The Meathead Manifesto.

Brody McVittie.

Foreword

This is advice for guys.

Guys who workout as hard as they party.

Guys who know what the 'Mr. Olympia' is.

Guys who subscribe to *Flex*.

Guys who know 38 variations of the chest press;

Guys who are probably clueless when it comes to women.

Guys like me.

When I was asked to write a series of bodybuilding articles for a renowned fitness website, I was thrilled.

Pumped.

I could do this in my sleep—and the result of that series, more or less, makes up *Book 1: Meditations on lifting heavy things, (many times in a row.)*

There's advice in there for everybody, but be warned—if you don't know your *'Dexter Jackson's* from your *'Branch Warren's*, you're gonna need Google nearby.

Bearing that in mind, the message is for everybody who ever wanted to get the most out of their time in the gym.

When I was asked to write a series of relationship advice articles for a popular Toronto lifestyle website,   *I.*   *Was.*   *Terrified.* Bewildered.
This was harder than seventh grade math—which was, coincidentally, about the time of my last mature, meaningful relationship.

I fooled my editor, though, and the articles contained in *Book 2: Meditations on Girls, and stuff* are the result of countless failed conquests with dozens of disappointed women.

When I was asked to write a series of articles on Nutrition, it was by *me.* To fill out the contents of this book.
I was pretty happy about it.
Bear in mind that I'm not a certified nutritionist— I'm just a guy who took an interest in building muscles, and the science behind feeding them.

Book 3: Meditations on Nutrition...and Supplementation (...and other stuff I'm grossly unqualified to give advice on) pretty much shares everything I've stumbled upon up to this point.

As a Certified Personal Trainer, I want to help my clients reach their fitness goals. As a writer, I want to give people the knowledge (and, hopefully, some motivation) to take their physique to the next level.

I know I'm trying to, everyday.

Hopefully, if you're reading this, you can learn something from this meathead's mistakes.

Table of Contents:

Book 1: Meditations on lifting heavy things, (many times in a row.)

Book 2: Meditations on Girls, and stuff.

Book 3: Meditations on Nutrition...and Supplementation (...and other stuff I'm grossly unqualified to give advice on.)

The Meathead Manifesto, Book I

Meditations on lifting heavy things, (many times in a row.)

Getting Through That First Week

…

So you took a chance, joined a gym.

Great.

You should know, there's more to it than flashing the pass on the end of your keychain; you're paying the cash, you better get in there, tough guy.

Sure, it's scary the first time. The lights are bright, the girls are beautiful and the *guys* — well, for every average-sized one walking around, there's two that could give He-Man a run for his money.

And He-Man is a *big* dude.

Yeah, there are dumbbells with numbers higher than you remember there being numbers, and He-Man in the corner has been putting them up since you walked in the door, but don't worry, little man.

There's a place for you in the free-weight room, and you better believe the monsters will respect you for getting in there and finding it, day in and day out.

Respect, a lot more than the guy peeking at you from behind the Smith machine.

…

Yeah, Mondays are tough, you tell yourself, but if cinnamon-skinned Sally can bust an hour on the elliptical, then you can get your lazy ass to the gym.

…

Sure, you injured yourself on the couch last night, but its Tuesday, and you know damn well Jack Bauer wouldn't hide from the Squat rack.

…

Wednesdays — well, Wednesdays suck for all of us.
Go to the gym.
Conventional wisdom states that you need an off-day; Thursday ain't it. The bench won't press itself, and you want to look pumped for the weekend, so Thursday might as well be Monday, because you're starting over.

…

By Friday, you've got to be feeling good — maybe good enough to smile at the walking L'Oreal commercial on the treadmill beside you — the one who's probably noticed your newfound *commitment*.

And not just because it's her favorite word.

…

Now, the weekend—the weekend could be your downtime. You could kick back; admire the hard work you've put in over the last five days.

Could—but you know damn well what Arnold would say, and Saturday is just two shy of Monday, so why ruin a good thing?

You're already the envy of the wimp hiding behind the Smith machine.

The Importance of the Training Partner

…

Okay, so you're a little nervous.

You've got every right to be—maybe it's been awhile, maybe you're worried you've still got some coleslaw on that dumb smile stretched across your face.

Relax—first dates are tough on everybody, superstar—just bat those pretty eyes, pick up the '35's, and curl 'em until your ears bleed.

It's your training partner's first time, too.

…

So what if he's got *zero* after the *two* on the measuring tape wrapped tightly against his arm?

Fourteen and a half ain't bad, and that fifteenth inch you're gunning for won't add *itself* to your bicep.

…

Working out with somebody new for the first time is hard on everybody, no matter if 35 pound dumbbells represent their max curl, or their bare minimum—but you can bet the best way to impress *Arnold* over there is to get on the bench, and just rep, coleslaw or not.

Because any bodybuilder worth his salt respects drive and determination over forced negatives and three plates.

Now, mind you, three plates aren't all bad, either, but the only way you'll get there is making the kind of call-in-sick-tomorrow lifts you'll need a spotter to cap off.

Think about it — nothing will make you feel better about adding that *third* plate than having someone there to share it with; someone who's been there for the times *two* almost broke you; the times *wife-beaters* were just bad dudes on the six o'clock news, the times coleslaw made you think twice about smiling at Sally.

…

So all you new meatheads, don't bother fixing your hair, and go say 'hi' to the monster trying to get his weight belt on. The worst thing that can happen is you walking away with an intimate knowledge of the mechanics of the Nike Deadlift Strap clasp.

Who knows — you could wind up with the single most important piece of equipment in that weight room — an extra pair of arms, twenty inches or otherwise.

…

And that—*that*—is worth all the coleslaw in the cafeteria.

What to Wear and (Infinitely More Important) What Not to Wear to the Gym.

As you've gathered by now, each and every gym (--or health club, or fitness farm; or whatever-the-marketing-guy-decided-to-call-it-to-hit-the-target-demographic--) is it's own delicate little ecosystem.

As such, the slightest imbalance can throw the harmony of the entire structure out of whack; madness, destruction and cataclysmic change can—and will—occur.

Take, for example, the sight of *you*—New Gym Guy—in a see-through mesh tank top.

It might have seemed like a good idea, winking at you from some forgotten corner of your closet.

Hell, you tell yourself, you've been making progress.

And the girl who does kettlebell training two benches down hasn't exactly noticed your ever-tighter fitting t-shirts, so, *logically…*

Don't.
Ditto the denim cut-offs, rainbow-striped workout pants, army boots, and the any-everything you wore to the gym the day before.

It doesn't matter whether you're rocking a body fat percentage in the single or *nowhere-near* digits; some things just do *not* belong on the male body.

And yes, your tye-dye shirt is one of them.

Be mindful of your surroundings; study the delicate eco-system you inhabit, and react accordingly.

If you belong to one of those yuppie micro-fiber-everything *because-sweat-isn't-really-an-option* cell-phone earpiece *so-you-can-conference-call –during-cardio* health 'retreat centres,'then, yeah, dust off the earpiece and be a tool too.

Conversely, if the boys over at Body Barn like to accessorize powerlifting chalk with their wife-beaters, it couldn't hurt for you to do the same.

Bear in mind that while, (by and large,) the majority of us at the gym are far too self-involved to notice *anything* you're doing, the fastest way to change that (and, in doing so, throw the whole damn eco-system out of whack) is to march in tomorrow wearing your spandex bicycle shorts.

How to Tell If Your Trainer Is a Douchebag

Fact: Personal Training is expensive.

Fact: The Fitness Industry attracts a great deal of mono-syllabic, knuckle-dragging Meatheads (--and by no means am I excluding the mono-syllabic, knuckle-dragging Meatheads of the female persuasion.)

Fact: Some Personal Training Certifications can be completed and issued over the course of a weekend; some Certifications literally can be completed in one's sleep. (As someone who has done both, I assure you this information is accurate.)

In order to protect your investment, here are some sure-fire tips to assure your Personal Trainer is, in no way, a Douchebag.

-Don't Be Oversold By Scientific Jargon.

Chances are, you'll have an opportunity to meet your Personal Trainer—usually free of charge—in order to hammer out the details of the torture (--in a good way--) to follow.

On the end of the trainer, it presents an opportunity to lay out what we sometimes refer to as your

'Periodization' program—a structured, professional breakdown of how and why you'll be hitting the necessary benchmarks en route to your ultimate goal.

This presentation should be researched, professional, and slightly over your head (--because, to be honest, if you knew how to replace the pistons in your engine head, you'd save money on labour costs *there*, too--) in that you're paying an experienced, qualified service professional for a result.

One you couldn't neccesarily accomplish on your own.

You know this—

The trainer knows this—

They don't need to beat you over the head with it.

See, any trainer worth their salt knows how to relate the association between Adenosine Tri-Phosphate and Lactic Acid Threshold (*told you) without appearing mysterious and aloof.

(*By the way, it's like this—the more you curl a dumbbell, the harder it gets, and the more it burns like hell…because you're exhausting the ATP and the Lactic Acid is the by-product.)

Having covered the goal from the trainer's point of view…

-Yours? (Or, Personality is Important)

Is this trainer a douchebag?

Seriously.

As a trainer, I could have a Master's Degree in Kinesiology, with a BA in Nutrition, and Certifications in everything from Senior's Fitness to Exercise Nutrition.

If talking to me is about as stimulating as conversing with the drywall in your bathroom?

It's never going to work.

No matter my qualifications, if I can't relate to you — if I can't get through to you — hell, if you don't like me — then me barking at you to lift something *slightly* too-heavy for you, *ten times*, is never going to happen.

Bottom line —

--you have to like your trainer.

Personalities meshing probably accounts for 80% of the successful client/trainer relationship. As I mentioned, you'll probably have the opportunity to sit down and game plan with your potential Personal Trainer.

Fortunately, I'm sure some psychologist (far smarter than myself) has established that you'll know 'within Five Minutes of meeting someone, whether or not you like them.' Meaning, ideally, you've got the rest of the hour/appointment to actually absorb the dumbed-down scientific process of the torture to come.

Yeah, you'll now really quickly whether or not you *like* your Personal Trainer, which leads me to my next point…

-Don't Judge Your Trainer by the Fit of His T-Shirt

This is the fundamental opposite of my first point, *Don't Be Oversold by Scientific Jargon.*

Just because your trainer shops at Baby Gap for his workout gear, does not make him a good trainer.

If your trainer's arms are the size of your waist, and you're looking to *not* have your arms be the size of your waist, always check his credentials.

On the other hand, if your goal is weight loss, and you look a hell of a lot more lean than your trainer, maybe they're not the ideal candidate to motivate you towards hitting those goals.

If your trainer's lats are so big that he can't turn sideways—if your trainer is developing increasingly-aggressive pustules over the course of your initial meeting—hell, if you have any indication that he got to that statuesque physique any other way than naturally—

    --run.

-Don't Judge Your Trainer by the Fit of Her T-Shirt

C'mon guys.

If You Happen to be 125lbs—and Your Trainer is 265lbs—and he's training You like *You're 265lbs*—Your Trainer is a Douchebag.

You'll know quick—on your very first session together, if he walks you up to a loaded Squat Rack, and, with a straight face, asks you to go "Ass-To-Grass" (*--all the way down, past 90 degrees parallel to the ground, Scientific Term--) with 300lbs?

Douchebag.

Hell, if he uses the term, "Ass-To-Grass," at all.

Ever.

Douchebag.

-Matching Energy

This oft-overlooked rule-of-thumb is just as important as making sure personalities mesh:

If you walk in for your four pm session, exhausted after a day of driving the kids to school/dealing with your asshole boss at work/ picking up the kids at school/ dropping off the kids at whatever-after-school-activities-they-need-dropping-off-at

AND THEN

showing up to be tortured (--in a good way!) then, yes, you want your trainer to be uplifting and refreshing and motivating. Not bouncing off the walls like they've ingested an eightball of cocaine.

The trainer is there to allow you to push hard and release some endorphins and feel *great-but-a-little-nauseous* and forget about the burdens of the world-resting-on-your-shoulders:

GIVE ME *TEN* MORE, YOU SNIVELING-MUELLING-DISGUSTING-SHELL-OF-A-MAN won't inspire.

Not one.

Certainly not ten, of anything.

Conversely, if you're ramped up to hit the weights hard (--like your workday--) and you catch your trainer falling asleep between sets, or texting, or snorting a line of the cocaine you now kinda wish he'd snorted ten minutes before you came in to workout, then, no, that's not indicative of matching energies, either.

A *'harmonious union of ideals, goals, and energies — synchronized and ever-progressing to said-goal's completion'* is the 'scientific' term:

All you need to remember is that it is important you're on the same page.

How to tell if you're a Douchebag Client

Fair is fair.

I've spent years on both sides of the Personal Training desk…I've been the dewey-eyed, farm-fresh iron virgin, and I've been the seasoned veteran who eats said virgins for breakfast (and cash.) So, as hard as I've been on my Personal Training Certified brethren, I'd be remiss if I didn't mention the shortcomings of some of our clients.

Hence, I present the following examples of who not to be when you invest in the expertise of a workout professional. I warn you in advance—as verbose and outlandish as some of the following stories may seem—they are (in fact and sadly) all true.

The Relentless Flirt

This one goes out to the ladies. Now, before you're quick to judge, please understand one thing—I adore each and every one of you. In fact, pretty much the entirety of *Book 2: Meditations on Girls, and stuff* details the fact that every problem, in every relationship situation, is the guy's fault.

Now, partly because I'm speaking from experience—and partly because you'll see why this just doesn't work the other way around—you girls are going to have to bear with me on this.

For God's sake, stop flirting with your trainer.

I get it. Unfortunately, in some situations, a woman will have absolutely no support system in her goals to feel, look and live better. There's the asshole husband who tells her she's too fat, and will *always* be; there's the control freak who chastises her for investing her money in a vision of her better self — there's even the guy who is so insecure, so petty and jealous that he secretly dreads the thought of his woman becoming 'more attractive' or 'more self-confident.'

A woman so used to these psychological, emotional and verbal beatings steps onto the gym floor, scared and hesitant and unsure, and she hires a Personal Trainer. All of a sudden she's realizing there's an inner-strength she forgot she had, and she's feeling better and she's looking better and

--and I'm all for, up until the point –

She realizes there's this young, ripped, gorgeous guy *(--it's my book, I'm allowed to build myself up a little bit)* cheering her on and complimenting her and believing in her in a way that no one else in her life is.

And then she's doing weighted back extensions one day, and she feels her trainer's sinewy (--because he's so jacked even his Goddamned *hand* is sinewy) on the small of her back (--because he's illustrating how she needs to break parallel on the concentric phase of the motion, in order to fully extend the muscles of the rectus Abdominis) and she feels a certain way about it.

And it's all downhill from there.

Now she *swears* it's *"because nothing fits right anymore,"* but she's showing up with more ass showing and she's specifically mentioning where she's meeting the girls Friday night *right after* asking where you're going when you mention you're going out Friday night also.

And she's making comments about her flexibility, and maybe she's making a few too many noises while she's straddling the abductor machine and she's asking for a cell phone number and when she gets it she veers from professional to unprofessional very fast and

--you get the point.

Don't be *that* girl.

The Over-Texter

Again, I have to clarify—the *Over-Texter* is a different animal than the *Relentless Flirt*. Whereas the latter has a clear, concise and calculated plan of attack, the former really, truly, has no idea what they're doing…and they're going to tell their trainer *All. About. It.*

They text before they cheat on their diet.

Standing across from ice cream freezer for last ten mins.

Weak.

Help.

They text after they cheat on their diet.

I texted you when I was in line but you didn't answer and there was a two-for-one and I was so hungry and why didn't you answer me I'm so fat

They text late at night.

Really late.

When they shouldn't.

When

Are you up I need you

Looks like

Are you up I need you

To whomever you're lying beside.

God forbid they start sending Selfies (*see all about it, *On Selfies & Sexting*, earlier) under the guise of

Look at your hard work

Or

Just a progress report

Or

This is what I look like naked.

You see how the *Over-Texter* can turn, very easily, into the *Relentless Flirt*? The gradient here is so steep, once the proverbial ball starts rolling, the classification between *Douchebag A* and *Douchebag B* is almost non-existent.

As trainers, we need to limit and enforce the amount of communication with clients outside of their designated sessions, thus limiting the dangers—and quantities—of bombardment. That hour per session, however, does little to save us from...

The Over-Sharer

Again, the *Over-Sharer* is a different animal—albeit with similar lack of respect for the professional boundaries between client and trainer—than the *Over-Texter*.

Whereas the latter is comfortable spreading the dump of uncomfortable personal information into any and all areas outside of their allotted training time, the former (while respectful of boundaries post-session) has a hell of a lot to talk about *during* that hour.

As a trainer, be prepared to weather storms like

My husband's lack of stamina in the bedroom

And

The green ooze seeping from my son's rectum

Amongst gems like

The effects my menstruation cycle is having on my ability and desire to allow you to do your job.

If you're thinking *"Hey, most of these traits and characteristics are remarkably similar,"* then you're absolutely correct. Professionalism is paramount—and present—on the majority of trainer/client transactions; illustrating the horrors potentially unearthed when lines become blurred, however, should help you make informed, concise and logical choices the next time you look into your trainer's eyes and think about sharing.

The Thing about Squats

Squats. Suck.

You know it, I know it, and — unfortunately — the dude with Will Harris wheels repping them out in the corner knows it.

He's doing them, and he doesn't need to.
You, on the other hand…

Manning up to leg day isn't easy for the *biggest* at the gym; for the rest of us, its murder. Unfortunately, bodybuilding is one of those 'get what you put in' clichés.
And every training article you've ever read wasn't lying when it told you that, hands down, nothing gives you a total body gut-check like spending time parallel to the floor.

So suck it up, call your mother to tell her you love her, and get under that rack.
There's things to consider, sure, when you line up your shoulders under the bar — whether or not you've upped your life insurance premium, how long it'll take for your girl to move on — really, though, the only secret to getting the dreaded squat right is actually *doing* it.

It doesn't matter if you're racking a plate a side or ten; as long as you're breathing right, tightening that Transverse abdominus, and dropping low, you'll have the respect of everybody around you for giving it a go.

And therein lies the magic—sooner or later, even if you've just got a naked bar draped across your delts—you'll find that 'sweet spot,' the point in the descent when you can feel your entire body say "THIS. IS. WORKING."

Going heavy isn't the trick; remember, a standard Olympic bar is forty-five pounds, and you're pushing all your upper body weight into your wheels when you work your way down.

Whether it's six reps or twelve, going full-bore and getting your ass parallel to the floor is all it takes to turn little-girl stems into the kind of proportionate-to-my-upper-body quads, hamstrings and glutes you (probably) so desperately need.

So the next time you see that rack free, pick up your cell phone, make the call, and give it a shot.

(A Little Bit) About Etiquette

Chances are, when you signed your membership contract, some gorgeous, in-shape membership-sign—up-person went over the do's-and-don'ts of the gym.

Chances are, you weren't paying attention.

The gorgeous, in-shape-*ness* of the membership-sign-up-person had something to do with it—
--but mostly, you figured you already knew the do's-and-don'ts of the gym.
(And if you didn't, you'd get the hang of it by the end of your first workout; common sense, right?)

You've got common sense—it's why you decided to get your ass in shape.

You *do* need to get your ass in shape.

You'd be amazed, however, at the number of common-sense *looking* gym members—and the number of them at your very gym—who have no common sense at all.

So for *those* guys (--and surely, you're not one of them, right--) here's one pretty basic/incredibly important rule of thumb.

Wipe the equipment down after using it.

Yeah, you've just hit a personal best on your bench press. You're straddling that half dead/feel like a million bucks line as you writhe your way out from under that barbell; either way, you feel both a little bit stronger, and a little bit *lighter*.

(You are.)

Because you've just left two gallons of sweat all over the bench—the bench you're now walking away from.

The bench the *next* guy who wants to hit a personal best on is looking at, disgusted.

To avoid a barbell upside the head (and, subsequently, heading to the Pec Deck only to discover that it, too, is soaked) take a second and wipe the equipment down after finishing your sets.

It sets an example to the *other* new guys (--the ones without any common sense--) and ensures the next piece of equipment you approach will be similarly sanitized.

(Karma is a bitch.)

It seems simple, sure—and, given the amount of bodies that hold said barbells, or lie across said benches, you would hope it is common practice—and it very well could be.

Just do your part in keeping it that way.

The Benefits of Circuit Training

You've heard its benefits praised in the change room of your gym; you've peered through the glass in the Personal Training Studio, seen the tolls it has taken on the fittest of the membership.

What the hell is Circuit training, and, more importantly, why the hell would you want to subject yourself to it?

The What

If nothing else, Circuit training is time-efficient. As a conditioning method, it is a resourceful way to combine aerobic fitness and strength training (-- admittedly, with less intensity than either modality if performed alone.) A common Circuit may consist of 15 reps or 30 seconds of 10-12 weight exercises, for both the upper and lower body.

The Who

Adopted and perfected by military divisions and sports teams, Circuit training benefits anyone looking to improve body composition (show) or stamina (go.)

The How

Strength

Now, the weights lifted during a circuit are usually 40-50% of a 1RM (one rep-max, remember?) or, literally, about half of what one would normally lift for each exercise. Alternating between upper and lower body exercises (so the arms rest while the legs work) while maintaining a steady heart rate is key.

Traditional strength training uses higher intensity loads and larger rest periods—usually 60-90% 1RM with 1-4 min rest. Studies have shown that blood lactate levels increase dramatically with Circuit training, suggesting a high anaerobic content to training.

Simply put, stamina—and the ability to tolerate elevated lactate levels (the dreaded burn) will improve.

Cardio

On average, one can expect heart rates of about 80% Max, but oxygen levels are only at 40% of maximum training capacity, which puts circuit at the minimum level for aerobic fitness improvement.

Therefore, Circuit training is considered low-to-moderate aerobic training, with benefits substantially smaller than meat-and-potatoes cardio. However, by dropping rest times between circuits, stimulus on VO2 max is accelerated.

For example, if you were to run at 75% of your maximum training heart rate for 20-30 minutes, 3x per week for 8-12 weeks, your average VO2 max would increase by 20%--in circuit, you would be engaging 80% of your Max THR.

Will Circuit Training get me Ripped?

Yes.

Research shows a 2.2-7lb gain in lean body mass (muscle) could be achieved—meaning one could expect a decrease in relative fat mass of 1-3%.

 Now, one's total weigh may remain unchanged; but, let's be honest—

--when you're on the beach, no one cares what the scale says.

The Final Word

Circuit training is better suited for toning than losing a ton of weight; for improving endurance and stamina rather than building raw power and strength. When implemented in rotation with weeks of a more sets-and-reps based training style, one will notice a substantial increase in energy reserves and, (--as a result of the activation of perhaps-previouslyunengaged stabilizer muscles —) a translation to more power when reverting back to strength training.

Debunking the Myths Surrounding Personal Training (+Training a Meathead!)

Fact: Personal Training is expensive.

Fact: You've got misconceptions about just what-the-hell your Personal Trainer does. (Unless, of course, you've invested in a Personal Trainer in the past—in which case, you're probably sitting on a beach somewhere, completely *jacked*, and fondly remembering the time you weren't, and you too had misconceptions about just what-the-hell your Personal Trainer does.)

Our industry seems to be the only one whereby one assumes that having a gym membership guarantees us the results we obtained said-gym membership to achieve.

Sadly, paying a forty-dollar-per-month access fee doesn't mean you can half-ass it three times per week and expect to lose the ten (*--okay twenty--*) pounds you swore to lose when you signed on the dotted line.

Think of it this way: if I need my engine replaced, would I go to my mechanic and say "Hey bro, I need to fix my engine, but rather than hire you to do it, I'm going to rent that bay over there for an hour, use your tools, and do it my *damn* self?"

Many trainers spend yeas training themselves, obtaining Kinesiology degrees from world-class Universities, and maintain aggressive yearly certifications—does your fitness know-how really supersede theirs?

No?

Then maybe it's time to stop dreaming of achieving your goals, and actually start achieving them.

Training a Meathead (Or, Why we bother to become Personal Trainers, at all.)

Fact: If you're a male, and you're reading this, and you've ever done more than three sets of something in some gym somewhere, then you think you know everything there is to know about fitness.

So, fact, you don't need a Personal Trainer.

Fact: You're a fool.

In order to break through plateaus, in order to achieve sport-specific advanced conditioning—hell, in order to be able to play with the grandkids one day—you need dynamic, aggressive, evolving exercise modalities.

Meaning, *no*, that shoulder routine you've been banging out for the past six months (--with nothing to show for it, other than that nagging rotator cuff injury) isn't as effective as you think it is.

No, just because you can make it another thirty seconds on the elliptical without falling flat on your face doesn't mean you're ready for the Boston Marathon.

You need a quantifiable *plan* — one that incorporates dynamic and static flexibility modalities, as well as specific, individualized aerobic and anaerobic system programming, and, most likely, a radical diet overhaul.

But hey, you've got that covered, in between work, and the wife, and the golf, and the kids, and the kid's soccer practices, and fixing Dad's back deck next weekend, right?

Think of it this way: That athlete you admire? The one with the sixteen abs, and the sleeve tattoos, and the *$85-million-in-endorsement-deals –just-because-he-looks-phenomenal-without-a-shirt-on*?

He has a Personal Trainer.

Why not skip the science of it, *stay* busy, and have that hour to *not* worry about what the hell to do after your bench-press? Allow someone who really knows what they're doing to worry about exercise selection, and just take the ass-kicking they're giving you.

Your favorite movie star does it.

Even for the most meat-headed of us, it boils down to our base, guttural need to compete…to be *better*…

If I'm barking at you, pushing you past your potential and telling you to give me *ten* more??

You'll get ten, come hell or high water.

If you're on your own, and you're moderately sure that the guy on the bench next to you is watching you, and you're moderately sure that what you're about to lift is more-than-moderately too heavy?

Maybe *six* will do.

Note the difference.

Form. Is. Everything.

You cheat.

Whether you admit it or not, there's that exercise, for *that* body part—the one you just can't get down pat. Right?

I don't care if you call it a Romanian Deadlift or a Turkish Get-Up or the dreaded squat; there's that one that lags behind, the one whose motion never feels quite natural.

(Lat Pulldowns, I'm looking at you.)

That exercise you can never push (or pull) quite enough of whatever-your-weight is on; the one that threatens to defeat you each and every time you see it on the docket for the day.

So you belly up to the bar, content on telling yourself today is the day it's going to be different, and you load whatever weight you think you can move on. (*Hint—it's too much.)

And for the next six or ten or *however-many-you-think-you-can* reps, you suffer your dignity and your form (--but not your pride!) and you move that damn weight.

And you cheat the whole time.

It's an ego thing — maybe two weeks ago, you moved said weight, your form only *kinda* pathetic.

Then again, maybe kinda pathetic was two *years* ago, and you can't admit that you're not as functionally strong anymore.

There's hope for you yet (provided you haven't thrown your back out swaying violently with each pull on the Seated Row machine.)

Tighten that *TVA*.

Incorrect form regarding the *Transverse Abdominus* (layman's terms — low-back-ish) is probably the single most neglected aspect of proper exercise execution.

By 'rounding' or 'swaying' the back, in order to add a little more kinetic chain (technical term: *uummph*) into a motion, it is the area we tend to be hardest on.

We, as human beings, tend to lift with the back, instead of the legs — think of the motion you use when getting up from the office chair, or out of the car.

Chances are, you're not using your quads, hamstrings, glutes and calves — chances are, you're not engaging your TVA.

To engage this musculature, essentially I want you to point your chest towards the sky — hell, try it right now.

(I know, I know — it's hard to tear your eyes away from my riveting pearls of wisdom.)

There.

Notice how your scapular set (layman's terms: shoulders, genius) automatically depresses and retracts?

This positioning is crucial not only to proper exercise execution, but it forces the spine into correct postural alignment as well. (Layman's terms: down and back is good.)

You should feel tension in your low back (--and, for a change, *good* tension, not that *I've-really-screwed-it-up-this-time* sensation you usually get after lifting something you shouldn't.)

This means you've engaged your Transverse Abdominus — which, in turn, means that you've extended and engaged the muscles surrounding your core (layman's terms: abs) which, in turn, is how you should hold yourself each and every time you toe up to a squat rack.

Or a Lat Pulldown.

Or a Seated Row.

Or a Military Press.

Or, seated as you are, while you read my next point.

(So) Breathing. Is. <u>Really</u>. Everything.

It's common sense.
As I've previously established, you're a meathead.
You don't have any.

So, yeah, I've been guilty of this myself—and, unfortunately, if you start this bad habit early, it is one of the absolute toughest to break.

Picture this: Chest day.
You're finally ready to put up that 225 on the incline bench for reps. (I didn't say it was necessarily the most *realistic* thing you've imagined yourself doing, but you'll get there, Superman.)

You're under the bar.

You've found that groove in the barbell your fingers love so much. (You know the one.)

You know you've never repped out eight of these bad boys before; you may have never even *wanted* to. Still, your spotter is a beast, and *'anything he can do, you can do—'*

Right?

So you pray to *whoever-you-pray-to*, you grimace *extra* hard, contract every muscle fiber in your chest/anterior deltoid/bicep/triceps/jaw/rectus Abdominus/sphincter/teeth (--just seeing if you're paying attention--) and you lift.

Suddenly, it's just you and 225.

(And, hopefully, the beast who is your spotter; chances are, even if he's directly behind you, at this moment, he's a million miles away.)

So you strain.
And you contract.
And you lower.

And you hold your breath.

*This, of course, is wrong, but hey: 225.

Point is, it's almost instinctual; for some of us, moments of great tension or anxiety tend to be somewhat *challenging* to our regular breathing patterns.

225 is one of those moments.

Any bodybuilder/sculptor/shaper worth their salt learned long ago that, while this might seem like something worth doing *here*, rep one — by rep ten?

Downright detrimental.

There's blood vessels to rupture, heart palpitations to incur and barbells to *lift-the-hell-off* of chests; holding your breath is really not going to get you out of this any easier.

Not only that, but a spike in blood pressure and intra-abdominal pressure can actually cause *Valsalva Retinopathy* — a (ouch) hemorrhage of the retina.
Now, this isn't permanent, but it ain't pretty.
And you're doing this to look pretty.

So, best advice I can give is to relax (--relax, here, being a relative term--) and suck in as much air as humanely possible.
As the bar begins it's motion up, up and as-away-as-possible from you and your chest cavity, I want you to take a nice, big, peaceful breath *out.*

Big Bad Wolf style.
(And, hell, with that 225 up, you *are* kinda big and bad.)

Always remember to breathe *out* during the *concentric* part of the lift (usually when the bar is fighting gravity, and you're fighting to stay alive.)

Remember, like it or not, that bar is coming back down again; and, like it or not, rep *two* is a helluva long ways away from rep *ten*.

Breathe accordingly.

On Selfies and Sexting

I've addressed our rampant insecurities; I've touched on the undercurrent of self-loathing percolating below our collectively-Crisco-covered veneers. Therefore, I'd be remiss to overlook one particularly potent/powerful/dangerous by-product of our self-obsession:

'Selfies.'

Coined by someone infinitely younger and more clever, a 'Selfie' is a snapshot taken (usually on an all-too convenient mobile device) with the sole-purpose of distributing said masterpiece to some form of social media, some imagined army of social media slaves anxiously anticipating

"Just me"

Or

"Grumpy"

Or

"Pensive at the Dollar Store"

Or

Whatever-The-Hell you label it.

It's douchey, almost delusional to perceive any one cares what you're doing At-Exactly 2:35 Easter-Standard-Time — so imagine the delight of your average meathead at discovering the power of the Selfie.

Biblical.

As bodybuilders, all we do is micromanage, catalogue, and compartmentalize our progress — every triumph quantified, every failure agonized over.

…And now we can share all of this?

Look around your local BodyBarn, and catch a trainer showing his client a 'most-muscular' pose from his last competition.   You know, not because he's oiled up and hard and impossibly dehydrated and granite-jawed — oh no, he's simply illustrating the need to bring out the lateral head of the triceps brachii in their workout, too.

By having archived records of our outright-dominance, all we're doing is justifying our need for constant, instant gratification; having someone else tell us how beauty-or-beast we are takes the pain away from chasing perfection, if only for a moment.

And then it's on to the next set, rep, series — and, now, dangerously, onto the next series of widely-available and always, in retrospect, embarrassing Selfies.

Which leads me to my next, extra-douchey subject: if Selfies are proverbial gateway drugs—then the next logical step to your average, Type- A Narcissist bodybuilder...

...outright Sexting.

Sexting: All Kinds of Wrong

For those of you decidedly less relevant, sexting is the act of "sending sexually explicit messages and/or photographs, usually between cellphones." Literally, an amalgamation of one of every meathead's favorite things

Sex

and one of his most-loathed

Texting.

(*Also known as 'pretty-much-anything-except-working-out.)

Sexting, naturally, was invented by a woman, as it remains the only reason we men look forward (--as in literally-foaming-at-the-mouth) to that otherwise-annoying *ping* telling us you're communicating.

Despite the overwhelming, all-encompassing risks associated with sending an image of one's penis to anyone else, the incredibly self-proud bodybuilding community has been quick to adopt this morally questionable social behavior.

Really, the only thing better than a standing-front-double-bicep?

A standing-front-double-bicep, *with penis.*

Catalogued and recorded and shared, because, let's face it: we weightlifters are delusional enough to believe that you're awestruck at the symmetry and power apparent in our latest Selfie:

The only way to send a picture so powerful—so revelatory—so senses-shattering that you're unable to maintain composure—hell, consciousness?

Yeah.

Somewhere along the way, we fooled ourselves into thinking that, despite the granite-chiseled perfection in our physiques, we could hold a candle to the nubile suppleness of the fairer sex.

We were wrong.

Now, for the female sexting sect, a warning as well: At some point in your lives (--no matter how inconceivable--) you're going to gracefully distance yourself from the life-of-the-party you are now. You're going to drive a minivan—a minivan full of the precious-little-angels you swear right now you'll never have—to various soccer games and band practices and school plays.

At these soccer games and band practices and school plays will be other precious-little-angels and their parents: parents who are now tech-savvy enough to have googled you.

Suddenly, that come-hither bathroom shot starring you and some strategically-placed Ready-Whip—or the spread-eagled-anatomy-textbook-grade photo of your vagina (--you know, the one you sent to that asshole who then dumped you and posted it all over the internet--) aren't such good ideas.

For every one of your son's sleepovers, forever, you're *that* mom to all of Billy's friends.

Guys, take it from every politician, ever—no matter how proud you are of your penis, it's not half-as-impressive as the most impressive penis she's seen. This bone-chilling realization hurts now: it will save you some shred of dignity in the latter years of your life, when shreds of dignity and sagging skin where your abs/empire used to be, are just about all you have left.

Better still than having photographic proof you're not the champion you used to be.

My Love Affair with DOMS

At first, my girl was worried. She said I talked about her every time I came home from the gym; said I wasn't careful with my verbose descriptions — hell, she admitted she was getting jealous.

I told her I was in love with DOMS.

She figured that new afternoons-and-weekends-trainer had a cute nickname, short for *Dominique* or *Diana* or something that started with *D* — you can imagine her relief when I told her it wasn't another woman I'd fallen for.

It was DOMS —
--Delayed Onset Muscle Soreness.

If you've spent any kind of time in the weight room, you know what I'm talking about. That burning, aching, cramping soreness in your muscles the next day, the kind that lets you know you really broke that muscle down.
You kind of become addicted to her; suddenly, a Tuesday morning without that intense tingle in your biceps means you must have failed in your arm training the day before.

Some scientists (far smarter than me) attribute the onset of DOMS to micro-damage that occurs to muscle tissue following those make-your-mother-cry workouts. It's one of those 'good pains;' the pretty cousin to that wicked-burn lactic acid — you know, the one that comes your way in the middle of that last set of curls.

I leave the science stuff to the egg-heads — all I know is that DOMS loves me, and I love her right back.

She's honest with me, DOMS is. (In ways I sometimes wish my girl would be after shopping for 'a few things' with my credit card.)

She lets me know when I've turned her on, and she's not afraid to tell me when I need to step my game up. I listen to her, and, in doing so, learn which areas of my workout I need to focus on in order to bring her howling back.

When she goes away, I chase her — only instead of buying pretty things to woo her, all I have to do is hit those seated rows again.

She knows how to give me just enough; after leg day, I'm not bed-ridden and miserable, but I'm not taking the stairs two-at-a-time, either.

If all my relationships were as mutually beneficial, I'd probably be a much happier man. For now, though, I remain content with my girl — she's got the out-of-the-gym stuff covered — besides, my thing on the side is always waiting for me after the squat rack.

The Rules of Attraction (--and Attracting--) At Your Gym

So there's *this girl* at your gym.
Am I right?

Maybe she's a regular at Sweat Yoga, maybe she's a monster on the treadmill, maybe (--but hopefully not—) she routinely presses more than you. Either way, you've noticed her, and you've noticed the shorts she wears when she's *not* noticing you.

Which is pretty much everytime you work out.
You want to know what you can do about it.

Let's face it, fellas; if you're staring at her while she hits the elliptical, chances are every other testosterone and NO-fueled meathead in the club is too.
Chances are Dexter Jackson doesn't work out at your gym.
Chances are somebody who *looks just like* Dexter Jackson does.
And if *he* can't get this precious little thing's attention, what chance do you have, right?

Wrong.

It's all about tact; you need to have a plan; you need to stick to it.

First and foremost, you need to be aware that there are essentially two types of girls who work out at the club. The first type—and sorry, boys, this is the overwhelming majority—want absolutely nothing to do with you.

This is a problem, because these are the types of girls you *want*.

The second type—and you can spot them a mile away—may be a minority, but they make up for a lack in numbers with their overwhelming sense of...being *overwhelming*.
Call them *gym-bunnies*, call them *easy*, call them *anything*—but don't *call* them. Because no matter how *Diesel* you think you are, there's always somebody a little more *Vin* right around the corner, and you can bet your sorry ass they'll be on to *them* by the time *leg day* rolls around.

So how do you separate yourself from all of the other available alpha males in your concrete jungle?

You try something so foreign, so alien--so unheard of—that she can't help but be intrigued.

You be yourself.

Not the guy you *think* she wants. You have no idea what the hell she wants. You're a man.

Not the guy with the biggest arms in the gym.

Trust me; you're not the guy with the biggest arms in the gym.
Not the guy who never does cardio, but hops on the stationary bike beside hers everytime she gets on. She knows you don't do cardio. You *look* like you don't do cardio.

No, the magic is in not being creepy; not hounding her by the smoothie bar, not trying to get her attention by lifting something you have no business lifting. (She can tell.)

The truth is, there is not set rule on *where* or *when* to make your move (—although when she's grunting through a set of shoulders may not be the best time--) just that if you do, for God's sake, be respectful.

Be honest.

Be yourself.

Put the Damn Weights Away.

What you were lifting wasn't that impressive anyway.

That, and you're helping contribute to a cleaner facility; there's nothing worse than crawling away from the squat rack only to realize you'll be spending the next twenty minutes unloading plates from the leg press—when all you wanted was a couple of quick finishing sets.

Chances are, if you're dedicated, you'll be hitting the gym at about the same time, on every training day.

That's great news—but you'll realize that the most dedicated guys—the guys in there at the same time as you, everyday—are also usually the *biggest*.

So if the monster next to you finds it's becoming a habit to clean up after you and your little sets of shoulder presses, there's a good chance he's not afraid to confront you about your lack of gym etiquette.
Better to take it from me, and never give him a reason to invade your personal space.

You paid all that money for your membership; you want to be able to show your face in the gym.

Finding Your Motivation

Maybe you don't look like Arnold. Maybe you don't want to.

Maybe you're more of a Steve Reeves fan — that old-school, farm-boy Hollywood physique.
Then again, maybe you thought Brad Pitt in *Fight Club* was about as good as a body could get.

Regardless of your aesthetic, chances are you've seen some dude on the street, or the squat rack, or the screen that made you feel a little…out of shape.

There's no shame in admitting that those quads are working for *him* — and there's no shame in using it as motivation to get your sorry ass back in the gym.

It doesn't make you weird or weak to admit to yourself that somebody else out there is rocking the look you want to.
Rather, it can be healthy — an ideal, a goal, a target. Whatever your motivation may be, finding it could be the key to kick-starting a stagnant workout routine.

We're competitive creatures, after all — say you haven't seen *Johnny from Accounting* in three months, and then he kills you on the squash court.

Not only are you utterly humiliated from the ass kicking, but your scrawny frame is winded halfway through, and the only tired thing about Johnny is watching his Polo try to hold in his *triceps*.

Rather than going home and bitching about how his macro-diet and split-routine is giving him an unfair advantage, why not spend five minutes getting him to detail his theory on pyramid sets?

Or, the next time you're watching a Stallone double-bill on the Action Channel, and your girl
(*--if you're fortunate enough to have a girl who'll watch a Stallone double-bill--*) can't shut up about how *cranked* he is, hop online during commercial and download his *Rocky III* workout program.

Trust me, she'll find *that* sexier than you complaining about how many *D-Bols* he must have been on.

Remember, the first step towards getting the kind of body you've always admired is telling yourself you can *have* it.
There's no great secret formula, no concoction of pharmaceuticals (--well, for the most part, anyways;) no magic wand to wave that gave your favorite star the physique they parade around your living room on   movie   night.

They simply wanted it, and worked for it.
You say you want it too--

--what are you willing to do for it?

Shut Up.

There's a dude at your gym — he might even be there *right now* — who thinks that screaming at the top of his lungs (every single time he reps an arm curl) is the thing to do.

That dude at your gym better not be *you*.

I don't care if every muscle fiber in your body screams in agony as you lower yourself under that next rep.

You keep it to yourself.

I don't care if you're moving the kind of poundages that make lesser men cry (--and don't even get me started on how *not* okay it is for you to cry at the gym--) you suffer in silence.

I don't care if the strain has caused your ears to bleed; I don't care if you've bitten clear through your tongue or ground your teeth down to the roots — you do not cry out.

Because, as earth-shattering and all-encompassing and awe-inspiring as your new personal best may be, the guy next to you doesn't give a damn.

That, and there's a very good chance that (while to you) the mountains of weight you're moving are impressive, they really don't warrant you howling like some wound-up simian each and every time your mouth moves as you move *them*.

Remember, as big as the dumbbells you've unracked may be, there's a dude two benches down moving *more*.

And if he's not two benches down, then he's on his way in from the parking lot—and when he gets here he really doesn't want to hear you making more of a fool of yourself than you most likely already are.

Getting Back Into It

Maybe you're not a beginner anymore.
Maybe you haven't been for years.

Maybe you've surpassed your expectations, maybe you've competed; maybe you've made it just about as far in the Bodybuilding game as you could ever dream—

--and then maybe you blow your knee out.

Injuries are part of the sport—any sport—and hardcore lifters know the perils of a torn ACL, or a rotator cuff, or quad; really, the possibilities are endless, and they're only *one bad rep* away.

For the dedicated, there really is nothing worse than watching weeks, months—*years*—of progress flushed down the drain. (And let's face it, there are only so many times you can watch *Pumping Iron* on the couch before you're clamoring to get back in the gym.)
So, maybe you've been off for a while.

Maybe that rotator cuff is where it should be, and you've reached that glorious day when you can get your skinny ass back in the basement.

Problem is — in the months you've been laid off — and whether or not you've noticed any substantial decreases in mass and definition — you just feel defeated.

Like all that hard work is gone —
--like it will take years to get your strength back to where it should be.

All of a sudden you're procrastinating; *'I've got laundry to do,'* or *'The kids will be home in three hours,'* or *'I'll get a good rest today, and crush it tomorrow.'*

Problem is, tomorrow is Tuesday.

And Tuesday is filled with excuses.
The best thing to do, tough guy, is realize that it took guts to grab the '45's in the beginning; back when you were a bodybuilding *nobody*, back when you were even *less* than you perceive (—and, probably, incorrectly —) you are now.

Weightlifters are, by definition, an anxious lot — every quarter-inch scrutinized and measured and catalogued; every new cut or line or vein a cause for celebration. Simply by realizing, *'Hey, I've done this before'* and grabbing those dumbbells (—trust me, your body won't care if they're '45's or '5's —) you're taking that all-important first step.

The step from the couch, to the bench.

Besides, you've seen *Pumping Iron* enough to know that (Spoiler alert :) Katz isn't going to find that T-Shirt.

Study up.

Studying. Sucks.

Maybe worse than *squats* suck — and we all know squats. Suck.

The thing is — squats *work* — maybe more than all other exercises put together, and that is why they're a staple of the every bodybuilder whose picture you admire in every bodybuilding magazine you buy.

Guess what else works?

Chances are, if you're reading this, you take *time*. Time in the gym, busting out your routine (-- hopefully, it includes squats--) time in the kitchen, slaving over egg-whites and sweet potatoes — time committing yourself, one-hundred percent, to the sport and the science of bodybuilding.

Chances are, you're set in your ways — back & bi's, chest & tri's — and who could blame you? If you've seen any kind of results with 'the way you do things,' why change?

Why study?

Because you can bet your ass the guy in the magazine does.

As mentioned, there is a science to bodybuilding. An ever-changing science—hell, break out one of your magazines from five years ago; I guarantee *half* of the nutritional and training recommendations have been revised or outright *revoked* in your latest edition of the same publication.

The reason is simple: competition.

Every year, new companies, supplements—new bodybuilders—are vying for their time in the proverbial spotlight; a little *bigger*, a little *better*, a little *stronger* than the one before.
That pill, to make the striations pop—that amino acid chain, to better enhance whey protein synthesis—that new exercise, to hit the posterior deltoid harder.

The great thing about all of this rampant competition—boundaries are broken and breakthroughs are made. *Everyday*. And all you—the new bodybuilder, the fitness enthusiast, or the un-converted spectator—has to do to take advantage???

Study.

Take it all in — be a sponge; absorb every relevant — *and non-relevant* — piece of information you can.
Study Dexter's posing routine, to see how he captured the 'O.'

Re-read Arnold's Bodybuilding Encyclopedia; see which exercises have stood the test of time, and which have been scientifically proven incorrect. (And yeah, the jury's still out on the *pullover-to-expand-your-ribcage*-thing.)
Discover why casein should be your go-to protein before bed — and read the article next month that tells you it *shouldn't*.

Be a student — admit that (--and this one's hard, fellas--) you don't know *everything* there is to know about bicep training, and that it couldn't hurt to hear some variations on the good-ol'-fashioned *curl*.
Who knows; your guns might thank you.

--And, if you can learn to admit that you don't know everything to your *girl*, I guarantee *she'll* thank you too.
(I realize that's asking a lot, but remember — Rome wasn't built in a day.)

Ask me how I learned *that*.

Knowing when to walk away

So you've been at this for a *while*.

Yeah, you know every variation of every exercise ever created—you can hit your upper chest sixteen different ways, and you've *forgotten* more about bicep curls than *Flex* could ever hope to know.

You're no longer a Bodybuilding beginner—you're the master.

Right?

Wrong.
You've got habits, is all—ways of training, ways of *approaching* training, ways of *thinking about* training. You've hit a plateau, and you don't even know it.

See, the moment you decide that you've learned everything there is to learn about Bodybuilding, you level out. You become complacent—hell, before you know it, you may even become disinterested.
In order to avoid this—in order to give your 'batteries' a chance to recharge, and, in order to realize that, *no*, tough guy, *you don't know everything there is to know*—
--you walk away.

Now, to any Bodybuilding enthusiast worth his squat rack, this is *murder*. After all, walking away means not training — *not* hitting those delts on Friday afternoon, *not* relishing the killer pump that comes only after the hardest of presses.

Walking away means sitting your ass on the couch, when you should be on the floor, repping it out.
Walking away is weakness.
Walking away is torture — walking away is *murder*.

And walking away might just be the best thing that ever happened to you.

Now, before you blow your fuse, you can relax — *this still is a Bodybuilding article after all* — and by no means do I mean you walk away forever.
(Because, again — to the hardcore — walking away=murder.)

You do, however, force your ass out of the gym — and into the park, or onto the beach — or yeah, the couch — and you take a little time off. Time off from training; time off from *thinking* about training.

Let your mind get excited about the idea of getting back on the weights; let your body ache for that pump—hell, let your head fool you into thinking that you're *shrinking* every single second you spend away from that crossover machine. (You're *not*—maybe in your time off, you'll stop being stubborn and actually *believe* those fitness articles that tell you *rest* is the key to growth.)

Trust me—by the time you're back at it, the pumps will feel better, the results will be better, and who knows—you might just view the whole Bodybuilding thing in a new light.

By some small miracle, you may even admit that, no matter how much of yourself you've invested—you're still, really, a Bodybuilding beginner.

And that isn't such a bad thing after all.

The Ladies' Only Section

It's the holy grail of your fitness facility.

The one place so tantalizing, so exotic, so appealing in its all-encompassing mysteriousness, that you would give all the protein shakes in the world just to be able to glimpse behind it's (probably) frosted glass doors.

The Ladies' Only Section.

To a new guy like you, it represents that *mecca*; that oasis, forever just out of reach to *you*, the moderately motivated, *quasi-good looking only-slightly-shlubby* fitness enthusiast.

And it's gonna stay that way.

Because you have a penis.

Which is, ironically, the very reason you're so interested in the ladies' section in the first place.
Thinking with it (your penis) has you imagining that every single female behind those (probably) frosted glass doors is a *ten*; which, looking around you at your club right now, explains why you can't seem to spot anything higher than that *seven* over on the elliptical.

It's a gym after all, right?

Stands to reason that the ratio of *really-super-fit-super-motivated-super-sexy-women* here is much, much higher than wherever-the-hell you go to meet women.

It might not be *half* the reason you signed up in the first place — but it *factored*, didn't it?

So you stand there, staring at (probably) frosted glass doors, slack-jawed at the mouth of greatness.
Picturing the stretching mats (--the ones right beside the pillow-fight bed and the oil-wrestling mini pool-) filled to the brim with decidedly *liberal* co-eds in various states of undress foam-rolling one another while you're feeling even creepier than you look.

Good news: it's not as glamorous as you think it is.

Sure, there are beautiful women working out in there — there are beautiful women working out in there right now.

There are also beautiful women at the bus stop, the library, and the grocery store.

And they're there for a *reason*.

Get it?

For some of you, the social aspect of your gym is part of the appeal—the atmosphere, the familiar faces, the chance that you could meet a girl who could love you the way only your mother has managed to.
What you need to understand—to respect—is that while, yes, some of the ladies may have similar mindsets, there are a portion of women at your gym (--working out right now--) who are there solely to hit individual, private goals.

Women who, believe-it-or-not, would like to do so without being oogled by you.

So while you can rest assured there are no pillow-fight beds or oil-wrestling mini pools behind those (probably) frosted glass doors.

Just hard-working, motivated, successful, beautiful women.

Women who spend their time *working out*, instead of standing mystified at the mouth of their private section.

Women who, as a result, probably bench more than you.

Brody McVittie

The Adonis Complex

Admit it, Superman: you spend more time in the mirror than your mammy, your lady, and all your lady's friends *put together*.

And while they're making sure their hair falls just *so*, you're obsessing about everything *else*, aren't you?

Hell, that hair could be losing faster than the Lions on Sunday, and your follicles would be the *last* thing you scanned in your reflection.

No, you're obsessing about every inch — every gain, every loss (--perceived or otherwise) in every body part you crushed out in the gym this week.

The slightest change in the fit of the T-Shirt you threw on means that your *protein intake* is too low.

You're looking *deflated* in the mirror downstairs, so you run to the bathroom off the master suite to double check.

Because, hey, *the lighting in there is better anyway*.

God forbid you have to let out the belt a notch during a cutting phase; you'd never eat solid foods again.

…

The truth is, as bodybuilders, it's our job to measure. To scrutinize. To analyze and overanalyze every aspect of our training, nutritional, and social routines, and calculate how they maximize — or detract — from our potential in the gym.

Or, in other words, obsess.

It's our job to obsess.

About ourselves.

Sure, we could argue that we're looking at our physiques as a sculptor might look to a lump of clay (--lump, depending on your definition of '*your definition*') but in all reality, we're narcissistic creatures.

It's the price we pay, willingly, to emulate the physiques of others we've obsessively studied.

There's the argument that, on some psychological level, we suffer from a type of body dysmorphic disorder—a chronic mental illness in which we can't stop dwelling on flaws in our appearance—be they real, or imagined.

I mean, by definition, BDD involves obsessing over one's 'appearance and body image, often for hours a day.' I don't know about you, but I spend at least an hour in the gym, and for that hour, I'm sure as hell obsessing over my chest. Or my triceps. Or biceps.

Rinse, wash, repeat, given the routine I'm crushing out.

And then, of course, there's the hour before the workout; the hour I spend *imagining* the workout, licking my lips in anticipation—waiting for that glorious swell, that pump I *need* to get me through the afternoon.

Heaven forbid, if I have to go to the mall, that I'm not *cranked*.

And then there's the hour I spend (much to my girl's dismay) recounting my triumphs on the squat rack, or the chinup bar, or the bench press.

But I'm a bodybuilder, right?

It's not like I'm some waifish model, vomiting in the bathroom because my ass looks a tad large before a runway walk.

No,   *they've*   got   problems.

I'm a bodybuilder.

Different.

Right??

Stretching.

You don't it.

And if you *do*, then you don't do it enough.

It is, *bar none*, the single most important component of any decent workout regimen. Regardless of whether you're gaining or losing, shaping or building, no self-respecting program neglects both static and dynamic stretching.

Pre and post-workout.

Every.
Single.
Time.

I stress this, because it is the one aspect of exercise new guys tend to ignore—we're all bench, or all biceps, and generally with *little-to-no* warm-up time.

By incorporating a solid stretching program—even just five or ten minutes per day, you're increasing muscle-specific range of motion; picture lengthening the isolated muscle, (and subsequent connective tissue) and safeguarding your body from strains and muscle tears.

Below are the two stretching modalities; feel free to experiment with both the next time you hit the gym — preferably *before* you load up your first barbell.

Static:

Ideally, you're working to overcome your body's natural stretch reflex (--the automatic tightening of a muscle when stretched--) which, in turn, will allow the sometimes-stubborn tissue to coax corresponding joints into a greater range of motion.

Static stretching tends to involve gentle, gradual holds; working a specific joint (or series of) through a range of motion to a comfortable end point.
Shoot for 20 seconds per hold; relax for another 20, and then hit it again. (This magic number corresponds directly with the aforementioned natural reflex; after approximately 20 seconds, the muscle tissue will loosen up.)

Working to improve flexibility at a specific position doesn't necessarily translate to increased flexibility *outside* of said position; so, while it is effective and easy for just about every demographic at your gym, you're looking for something a little *more*.

Dynamic:

These flexibility exercises use ever-increasing dynamic movements through the *full* range of motion of a particular joint.

In English, this means you're furthering your range through the process of *Reciprocal Inhibition* — wherein the agonist muscle contracts, allowing the *antagonist* (opposite) muscle to carry through the lengthening process.

Hit these bad-boys right, and you're warming up the joints, maintaining your current level of flexibility, and reducing muscle tension, all at once.

You'll generally be moving at a snail's pace to begin, and ramping up both speed and intensity as you progress through the motions.

The advantage of incorporating dynamic stretching — particularly before hitting a series of squats (--or anything that involves a wide range of motion, speed, or explosive movement--) is substantial; practice daily, you'll be '*Ass-To-Grass*' (*full depth, *technical term*) under that loaded bar before you know it.

Example: Static

Sitting on the floor with your legs in front of you, bend forward at the hips (--keeping your spine in a neutral position--) and feel the tension in your hamstrings.

What you're doing here is, in essence, forcing your hamstrings to relax, and in doing so, you're increasing your range of motion at the hop joint.

(You don't want to 'flex' your spine, here—though you will increase range of motion of your vertebral joints, you're deceasing the effect on your hams.)

Example: Dynamic

Stand on one foot. (Easier said than done, right?)

Now flex the hip joint of your non-supporting leg (yes, that means the one in the air) by extending the knee, allowing it to move like a pendulum.

This motion contracts the hip flexors (agonists) and forces the inhibition or outright relaxation of your hamstrings. (Antagonists.)

Remembering the 'Little Parts'

We've all got 'em.

Little Parts — wrists, calves — maybe a deltoid or two. Parts that just don't grow — parts that we hate to train, because they don't blow up.

They don't pump.

They lag behind — worse, they make us feel like we're missing out on a great workout — (for some body part we *can* pump —) every single time we hit them.

So we *don't*.

Hit them, that is — and if we *do*, we don't do it as often — if we do, we don't do it as hard.

It's basic bodybuilding psychology, really; we focus on the muscle groups that make us feel good. The muscle groups that we know we can count on for results — the body parts we know will swell every single time we work them.

We're visual beasts, us bodybuilders — and we want to leave the gym or the basement or the club feeling like we've *accomplished* something.

We want to leave feeling like we *look* as huge as we're *feeling*.

Before we know it, a pattern develops—and before we know it, we've got *Little Parts*.

All of a sudden, they're staring back at us in the mirror—those imperfections, those flaws in-an-otherwise-flawless physique. They're holding us back, affecting our symmetry, our proportions—and, if we're blessed enough to get up on that stage—they're undoubtedly holding us back on those judges scorecards.

So, what's the fix?

The best advice (—for those of us cursed with *Little Parts*, and for those of us not yet *blown-up* enough to notice them—)is to incorporate them, wholeheartedly, into our workout routines.

It *reads* easy, sure; trust me, though—if you're developed enough *everywhere else* to have *Little Parts*, then you've developed habits of not training them in the first place.

So,

Yes, this means priority training.

Yes, this means looking like a fool wrist-curling five pounds.

And, yes, this means you're not always going to pump the way you would on a regular arms day.

Put in the work—

--convince yourself that you can catch those lagging calves up to your massive quads—

--and maybe—

--just maybe—

--you can make your *Little Parts* a bad memory.

Muscle Confusion

We're creatures of habit.

Over the years, we tend to develop routines; daily patterns, or motions we go through, often in an effort to alleviate the stresses compounded on us as we progress through our hectic lives.

The morning coffee we can't live without, the grocery store after work on Tuesday, getting the car washed before taking the kids to soccer practice, hitting on the hot girl's *slightly-annoying* friend before zeroing in on the *real* target.

Regardless of the pattern, chances are you've got one.

Unfortunately, this can extend to your workout regime—and that's a very, very bad thing.

See, the trick to gaining lean muscle--or shedding unwanted inches—is to keep your body guessing; to stay one step ahead of our wondrous ability to recognize patterns, and adapt.

It's easy (--given the zombie-like state you're undoubtedly in by the time you make it on to the gym floor--) to simply tell yourself that it's Monday, so *Chest Day*, and then go bang out three sets of bench.

Maybe the first six Mondays you break a sweat; maybe the first six Tuesdays you're a little sore.

You tell yourself you'll change it up *next time*; but next time you're in a bit of a hurry, and somebody else is on the decline bench, so just hitting the ol' flat barbell presses will have to do.

Hey, it's better than nothing, right?

Soon, *next time* is something you say *every time*, and every Monday, you're under the same barbell and, to make matters worse, the barbell is loaded with the same weight.

You're really not sweating anymore, and there's no DOMS Tuesday mornings, either.

You need to change it up.

The good news is 'muscle confusion' is a buzz-term that actually has a variety of (very useful) implementations.

It could be as simple as altering the selection of exercises — and the sequence — for the day's lifts.

Suddenly *'Chest-and-Triceps-Monday'* is *'Superset-Incline-Press-with-Incline-Flyes'* instead of three sets, ten reps on the flat bench.

Feel free to micro-manage with rep counts, sets and rep times — hell, any change 'counts.'

It could mean a whole new series of training modalities; moving into timed sets, circuit training, or even challenging your existing exercises with different equipment — be it kettlebells or resistance bands.

You might be reading this, thinking *'but I like my training program.'*

'Why change a good thing?'

The sum of training effect is why. The most commonly recognized real-life example of a body's adaptability to exercise is demonstrated by observing the fitness of postal letter-carriers.

Part of their gig involves walking hundreds of kilometers per week, often in less-than-ideal weather conditions.

Naturally, they're all super-lean and ripped, right? Actually, due to the fact that the stimulus never really changes, once their individual bodies become accustomed to the rigors of their particular routes, they plateau.

Without new stimulus to jar them into adaptive responses, those hundreds of kilometers per week are no longer viewed by the body as exercise; rather, they've become just another part of the routine — as natural as that morning coffee.

So the next time you've risen from the dead and made it into the club, remember that although it would be easier to stick to the routine, you owe it to yourself to change it up — you made it to the gym, you might as well get something out of it.

Who knows; maybe next Monday, and the Monday after — the you that shows up might still be a zombie…but a slightly better-looking, *fitter* zombie.

Intensity.

No other word will go farther in determining the kind of workout you're having.

When you're pushing through previously established personal limits, endorphins are being released, muscle fibers are being strained, Adenosine Triphosphate (ATP) is being spent, and, obviously, your heart is pumping faster than it was the last time you made eyes with the girl from the shake bar.

By calculating your ideal heart rate during exercise, you can take steps to ensure you're making the most of your time in the gym.

Your maximum heart rate is determined, more or less, by taking the number 220 and subtracting your age.
For example, a 30 year old meathead has a HRmax of 220-30=190 beats-per-minute (bpm.)
I stress 'more or less' as it is not uncommon for said 30 year old to have a maximum heart rate of as low as 180 bpm, or, conversely, as high as 220bpm.

Using this formula would then over predict the intensity for people with a low HRmax, and under predict the intensity of people with a higher HRmax.

As with everything else, this is merely an accurate estimation, and one that could be incorporated as a baseline.

So, having calculated your maximum heart rate, determining exercise intensity is simply a matter of percentages. (I know, math is painful for me too — but this will pay dividends in the gym.)

Folks far smarter than myself have determined that an appropriate range of recommended exercise intensity is anywhere between 55% and 90% of your max heart rate — this percentage is known as your *target heart rate training zone*.

Landing in this range will ensure you're working hard enough for cardiorespiratory gains — but not so hard that the aerobic system is unable to provide energy (--thus engaging your anaerobic training system.)

Apply this formula to bouts of aerobic training — hell, go for 75%-90% of your HRmax next time you hit the treadmill — and you'll be carving a new physique in no time.

Tough Love

Admit it — you love to hear you look good.
Its validation, isn't it? I mean, you put hours —
years — of your life into the gym, or on the stage;
always working, always *translating*, that image of
your best self in your mind, striving to force it into
reality.

You never quite get there, though — in your head,
your traps should peak a little higher, and there's
always that phantom inch you've been chasing,
always just slightly out of reach.

So you love it when your girl, your neighbor, your
buddy--or your buddy's girl — notices the strides
you've been making, the gains you have achieved. It
feels good; even if you're not the bodybuilder you're
aiming to be, you're solid enough to impress those
around you.

The problem is, sooner or later, if enough people tell
you that you look good, you believe them.

Don't get me wrong — positive reinforcement is
crucial to the bodybuilder's (admittedly fragile) ego.

We need to hear we're making progress, that we're
jacked, solid, lean — whatever.

The danger, however, comes when we begin listening to those around us—and using *their* perceptions of us as barometers of our progress.

Maybe you begin to figure you're already there—where you desire to be, physically—and maybe you take it easy the next time 'shoulder day' rolls around.

After all, *Debbie-in-accounting* said you looked huge at last week's company barbecue. And *Debbie-in-accounting* is never wrong.

See, I believe we need to *not* measure up to the image of our 'perfect' selves. It's the proverbial *carrot-on-a-string* dangled in front of us, driving us ever-onward, even when well-wishers and supporters have assured us the race is over.

It's fire, really—something deep down and innate and wholly personal.

It's fire that forced you to get off your ass and pick up a dumbbell in the first place; it's fire that makes you dust off those training trunks every time *since*.

The Meathead Manifesto, Book II:

Meditations on Girls, and stuff.

One of the guys

So it's Friday night, and, to be honest, I'm going out with the guys.
I look my girlfriend dead in her eyes, smile my '*I'm not lying*' smile, and then move the lips that smiled it.

The words that come out are all lies.

Well, not *all* — I *am* going out with the guys — but, we're not just going over to a buddies' house to watch the fight on Pay-per-view.

No, we're going to a club, and then another club, and then a gentleman's club — and even though we won't be getting into nearly the kind of trouble my ego pretends we could — even though she probably wouldn't care if I told her the truth — I look her in the eyes and lie on my way out the door.

Why?

I just can't help myself.

I am, after all, a guy.

And there are a lot of others who would do the same thing.

Or so I thought.

The truth is—no pun intended—there is some kind of macho-code among little boys as we grow up, hours on the playground puffing up our chests and boasting of not-quite-true exploits that we retain as we grow older.

Sure, we're not 'beating up a hundred guys' or 'kissing a hundred girls,' but we still, in our social circles, have some innate need to prove ourselves— often at the expense of another.

So, picture my Thursday afternoon, making plans for the aforementioned Friday 'guys' night,' and having to tell the boys that *no*, I can't make it, and because my girlfriend and I have an agreement that we don't go to clubs. (And then other clubs, and then gentleman's clubs.)

The boys would never let me live it down.

The kid on the playground I *used* to be would roll over in his grave.

We're brought up in a competitive culture, and, subliminally, we retain all of the desires and yearnings that acceptance—achieved through victory—obtain; therefore, if I lie to my girlfriend, and downplay the proposed 'puffed-chest' grandeur of the evening, I'll be accepted by my peers.

I'll be one of the guys.

Truthfully, we won't be 'beating up a hundred guys,' and there's no way I'd have the guts to even *talk* to, let alone *kiss* one hundred girls, but somehow lying to her about the vivid imaginations we've conjured for the night makes me feel it's possible.

The truth is—and I'm, again, being completely honest—the night came and went without beating up one guy, or kissing one girl. No, we went to a club, and then another club, and then a gentleman's club— and not one of the questionably-nutritioned girls made me think for a second about leaving my sweet little somebody waiting for me at home.

To make matters worse, my sweet little something found out (and it doesn't matter how) that I had lied about where I spent my Friday night.

Hanging my head in shame, I fessed-up during our little 'confrontation,' and, to my amazement, she wasn't angry about the club I went to, or the other club I went to, or even the gentleman's club I went to; she was disappointed I felt compelled to hold the information from her in the first place.

In her mind, this made every Friday night with the guys before — and every Friday night with the guys since, probably — the subject of greater examination.

Trust me guys, the seed of distrust is not one you want to plant.

(And go easy on me for the analogy — it's my first relationship article.)

It's funny, isn't it — the little boy on the playground, the one beating his chest and bellowing at the top of his lungs — isn't as dead and gone as the years tell us he is.

No, his name is *ego*, and he's *right there*, behind your ear when you're looking your girl in the eye, whispering for you to lie when she asks,

"Where are you going tonight?"
Honestly?
The *right* answer is the right answer.

For the taking

It starts small.

Maybe you're not feeling the run to the grocery store one Saturday, maybe you ask her to go for you. Maybe she does, and maybe the next time you need groceries, you don't really feel like going again.

Maybe you ask her again.

Before you know it, Saturday mornings you're rolling out of bed, and *expecting* her to be heading out to the Superstore—before you know it, you're taking her for granted.

Ladies, maybe your significant other has a way with his hands; he said he didn't mind fixing the dryer in the basement or the leak in the upstairs sink—why wouldn't he want to renovate your basement?

My point is, nobody intends to take their partner for granted. (Or, if you do, you're probably better off finishing this sentence and then breaking up with them right after. Trust me; you need to be alone right now.)

For those of us still here, the road to 'taking them for granted' is more of a steep, steep hill. It starts small, sure, but a successful result can lead to an assumption that the next time, the result will be the same. So one week of eggs every morning can turn into a *months'* worth of waking up expecting to smell the bacon sizzling next to it.

Don't feel guilty if you're reading this and realizing that damn, you expect bacon and eggs too—maybe the cook in the other room likes slaving over a frying pan for you. Just realize that the decision should be theirs and theirs alone—your influence, based on a habit, can have absolutely no bearing on their decision making process.

Maybe the next time, ladies, that the handyman you love so much is set to tackle the eaves trough cleaning, you surprise him by getting on the ladder first. (I strongly recommend you leave the heels off for this.)

Fellas, fifteen minutes out of bed could have you cracking eggs *instead*; trust me, changing it up for her could pay off for *you* later on.

We're creatures of habit, sure; having some routine in a relationship is necessary. I'm sure both of your lives are chaotic enough apart, and there is an appeal to knowing that you can look forward to dinner in front of the TV tonight. While that is all well and good, expecting to eat your chicken and rice in front of Seinfeld re-runs can drain the magic out of your moments together faster than Jerry saying something cynical.

So tonight, would it kill you to cook the bird yourself, and surprise them with candles and a meal at the table and a 'How was your day?'
Remember, it starts small.

You may find that changing it up — surprising them and reminding them that *no*, you don't take them for granted — can take something just as little.

It's only the payoff that's big.

Why Women Love Assholes

So you're an asshole.

You're about to pick her up for your first date, and you don't really know which way to play it. You know you should do the right thing, take her somewhere fancy. Buy her dinner—pull out the chair for her, hold the door, take her coat. Be *that* guy.

Except you're not *that* guy.

You're the other guy. The skip dinner, skip the awkward-fake-politeness—if you can make it out of date number one—skip meeting her parents guy.

The *take-her-straight-to-your-place* guy.
And you might be better off for it.

Sometimes—

--and fellas, this is only sometimes—
--sometimes it's better to just be yourself.

Sometimes it's better to be an asshole.

Maybe it goes all the way back to the first grade. Sure, Billy brought little Suzie dandelions everyday, but Timmy — Timmy with the curly hair and the baby blues — Timmy pulled Suzie's hair, and Timmy stole Suzie's lunch, and Timmy tattle-tailed when Suzie kissed him on the cheek at recess.

The point is, Timmy got kissed, and Billy got the shaft.

Women love the 'bad boy,' and it's not just because every favorite soap opera and every favorite movie and every favorite song have at least one. The idea of 'taming' him — accomplishing something that no amount of parental guidance or peer counseling or law enforcement can — appeals to the hopeless romantic in her.

Yes, the same hopeless romantic that wants you to skip that reservation tonight.

Now, there are limits as to just how much of an asshole you can be — changing restaurants on a whim is okay; playfully 'picking on her' over appetizers *somewhere else* might even be a good idea, but, if you do go out, don't be an asshole to the waiter. Don't make it obvious that the girl at table two is wearing her dress *well*.

Be an asshole, sure — but be *her* asshole.

'Controlled danger' is the term of the day; it means skipping the reservation, sure, but knowing that your favorite little place will have a table available — or, if you go 'full asshole' and take her right home, it means you've got a bottle of her favorite vintage on chill, and are damn sure you know how to cook that frozen lasagna.

Toss a little spice into the date by being unpredictable, rough around the edges and maybe just a little wild — but never, ever, make her feel uncomfortable, or anything other than safe when she's out — or in — for the night with you.

So pull up for that first date, and let her think she knows where she's going for dinner. Let her think you're the nice guy she secretly wishes you're *not*.

And then, little by little, give her the real you.
The asshole.
Don't take my word for it — just remember the story about little Suzie and bad-ass little Timmy in the first grade.

Then remember little Billy.

As a recovering asshole myself, I can assure you, we don't get many opportunities to present ourselves in a positive light. So, really, you're doing all of us out there a favor tonight, when you pull up, flash that smile, and let her in on a little secret.

Why men cheat.

You can try to blame it on that *nature* thing; the whole *'spread the seed,'* *'continue the line'* psycho-babble men (much smarter than me) have attributed it to.

Then, of course, there's that whole 'alpha male,' macho-man, 'go forth and conquer' mentality that keeps relatively sane men behaving like fifteen year-old boys.

The question, again —

--why men cheat.

The short answer?

Because, largely — and to a man--

we're fools.

We know we've got something *good* at home; the kind of good that has coffee ready every morning before work, the kind that does the laundry. The kind that –in a way that no other woman since mother *should* or *will* or would ever really, really *want to* —cares about every minute detail of our (probably) mundane, miserable little existences.

Yeah, *that* kind of good.

See, to them—the good, good girls waiting for us at home—we're Rockstars and teen idols and champions—and they make us feel so damn good about ourselves, that we sneak out on them Saturday nights, maybe because we believe we actually *are.*

Maybe we believe that we'll be just as fabulous to the *next* girl, the one we waste time hitting on in dive bars and restaurants, on Saturday nights better suited for cuddling on couches somewhere safe.

Naturally, the *next* girl doesn't care; she might, if we're 'lucky' for a night or a weekend or the amount of time girls-on-the-side spend *being* girls-on-the-side. Regardless, the memories and good times and trust we tarnish by disrespecting our women (who, more often than not, we leave, selfishly, alone waiting for us) is never, ever worth whatever we gain by cheating.

And yet we do it.

We cheat.

Why?

There's no magic answer, no universal truth or secret coda I can reveal—no 'man card' I'll lose if I were to give up the magic formula that makes us the idiots we are. All I can offer, as a cheater a time or two (or three) myself, is that we're selfish, spoiled, delicate little boys, often hoping to give our frail little egos a boost.

Naturally, I'm not speaking on behalf of every man (or even every cheating man) but I can honestly admit that as a reformed-cheat (and yes, we *are* possible out there in the wild) I've matured enough to abhor the concept of betraying any relationship I've deemed worthy to devote more than a passing moment to.

So, looking back, what's my excuse?

Surely, I must have blamed *them*—the good, good girls waiting for me somewhere *other* than the *wherever-else-I-was* when I cheated, right?
Wrong.
Like the act itself, I really had no reason.
I was happy in a relationship.
I was content.
And then this *other* girl walked by and looked my way...

I don't want to scare any women out there, but, really, there is no rhyme or reason as to why we do the stupid, selfish things we do. The only thing I can suggest—and this has worked wonders for me—is establishing the importance of honesty early and often in the relationship.

The kind of guy who isn't afraid—hell, the kind of guy who's proud—to come home and share every detail of a hard day, or tell stories of events that make him feel 'weak' or 'emotional' or 'defeated' (to a good, good girl who'll listen) speaks volumes towards maintaining a healthy relationship, one that fulfills all the needs he has or could ever have.

The *other* kind of guy, the guy with secrets and things he can't be bothered to say—that kind of guy you don't want anyway.

How to Win her Over (or at least get her to call you again.)

You're taking her to dinner tonight, Romeo.

Here's a few key things to remember on this, the potentially-most-important-date-you'll-ever-have. (Provided things work out.)

-Take her somewhere off the beaten path. The Keg is great, sure, but she'll think you're a man-about-town for discovering that hidden gem

-Establish eye contact early. You're confident, interested, and completely invested in every work that pours out of her precious little mouth. Prove it.

-Compliment her—but not in a creepy way. *"Your ass looks fantastic in that dress"* may not go over; try something a little more tactful.

-Don't dominate the conversation. She may want to hear about the company's latest acquisition over appetizers—if you're yammering on by the time the dessert menu hits the table, you're an idiot.

-Maintain eye contact. You're *still* confident, interested, and completely invested. Prove it.

-Actually, really care about the conversation. If you're not interested in her ambitions, career, previous experience and worldview *now*—then you're probably never going to be, and you're probably not that into her.

-Don't make a big deal about picking up the cheque. (And fellas, in this day and age, it's okay if you don't—either way, keep it discreet.)

-Chivalry isn't dead (--it's just on life support.) You're not an ass if you open a door for your lady.

-Make sure she gets home safe. This may mean holding off on the mojitos; then again, getting hammered in front of her on Date #1 is a pretty good way to ensure there won't be a Date #2.

-Don't expect that kiss at the door; hell, don't expect *anything*. This way, if it happens—if anything happens—you get to go home feeling like *the man*. If not, you're not a chump.

Finally, (as always) I sum it up like this: *be yourself*. Just *better*. (Or, at least, on your best behavior.)

And, as a parting gift—a little free information about Date #2—never, ever, act surprised that she let you take her out again. (If you treated her *half* as well as I've outlined above, she will.)

How to Win Her Back (--provided there's any winning back to be done)

So you've blown it. Again. Take a day to mourn the loss of the best thing you've ever had — take ten — and then get your ass off the couch, put down the tissue box, and use these tips to get her back in your life.

-Let her go. The warning signs were there, Romeo; she needs space. This is why she moved out on your ass in the first place.

-Give her time. Not too much — you don't want her to get over the relationship — but you need to respect her wishes, and you need to give her a chance to miss you. A week of absolutely no contact — especially if you lived together, or saw each other every day — is plenty.

-Call. Sure, you want to show her how strong you are; how you're not like the other ex-boyfriends who called out of the blue, using some lame melodramatic excuse for picking up the phone. And yeah, you want to prove you can get by just fine without her, but let's be honest — you're a goddamned mess.

-Don't call. Yeah, this contradicts the previous point, but bear with me. You should call her, sure, but you need to be very conscious of *when* you're doing it. Three-thirty in the morning, after spending hundreds of dollars (and crying on shoulders that would prefer you weren't crying at all) at some club is not the time to be pouring your heart out over the phone.

It will make you look like an asshole.

You probably are an asshole, which is why you're alone right now.

If you're trying to win her back, though, you really don't need to remind her of this fact.

-Text. I think the point I'm establishing here, is that the most important step you can take (after burning your relationship all the way down) is to *take* the first step. Don't wait for her, trying to be stubborn and foolish and proud; those are traits that landed you loneliness in the first place.

Now, by *texting*, I don't mean writing a book; keep it sweet.

Keep it simple.

'Miss you' will do just fine.

(If you have some cute pet name, or some saying that was strictly between the both of you, now is the time to dust if off.)

-Arrange a meeting. This, boys, is tricky; you don't want to seem overbearing, or lead her to believe that by meeting, you in fact want to sleep with her again.

You do.

She knows, and you know.

Better to leave it unsaid.

The trick to meeting her is *location*. Make it neutral, make it public; make it non-threatening. Somewhere she knows you won't have the balls to get into a screaming match about how 'unfair' she was to you in the break-up.

-Pull out all the stops. It's time, provided she agrees to meet with you, to remind her why she fell in love with you in the first place.

If your name is Tim, then you'd damn well better be 'First-date-Tim.'

If your name is Ed, then you'd damn well better be 'First-date-Ed.'

And so on.

-*Earn* your time with her. From here, guys, you're on your own. You were the one in the relationship; you know what works — and, by now — what clearly doesn't.

Take it easy.

Take it slow.

Trust me; if she was worth the trouble in the first place, then she's worth the trouble of winning back.

How to Survive the Post-Dinner Movie (Without Coming on Too Strong)

I'm making a couple of assumptions here.

I'm assuming you've been on a dinner date with somebody you want to get to know…a little better.
I'm assuming you're doing the tried-and-true 'dinner-and-a-movie' thing (--I refuse to call it a cliché—it's really more of a classic--) and I'm assuming you're clever enough to realize the stresses of a multiplex can't really compare to cuddling up on your (--or her--) favorite couch.

So, Romeo, you've done dinner, and you're fortunate enough to spend the rest of the evening alone together.

Here's how to NOT blow it.
-Rent something she's going to like. Let's face it— you don't give a damn what you rent. I don't care if you can get your hands on a bootlegged *Transformers* sequel—no matter how badly you've been waiting to see the latest release, you've been waiting to see her *naked*, even more.
(This isn't likely going to happen on date number one—she's a *lady*, remember—but you're a hell of a lot closer if the rental is something she can stomach.)

-Be subtle in inviting her home. You're going to suffer through *The Terms of Endearment*; the least she can do is let you suffer on your ottoman.

I'm with you; but be tactful, fellas. Don't come across as creepy—no maniacal grin with the invitation—throw it out gently, one of those *Hey,-I've-got-an-idea* ideas.

-It's called a *loveseat*, fool. Use it.

-Nothing is sexier—*nothing in the whole wide world*—than a bottle of red wine. The trick, again, is to make it seem subtle. If she walks in, and you've got rose petals all over the loveseat, and a bottle on chill on the table, then I'm afraid you're walking the 'creepy' line.

Some girls might appreciate the attention to detail, but the 'spontaneity' of the evening is part of the appeal.

-Let her watch the damn movie. This is the part that sucks, but you knew you'd be on the frontlines when you signed up for the war. There won't be a moment of the god-awful romantic comedy that you wouldn't rather be diving down her neck, but you're a gentleman. So you watch.

So you suffer.

-That said, if she makes the first move — and yes, she's still a lady if she does — then all bets are off.

-If the movie ends, however, and her (being a lady) and you (being a gentleman) has not led to ravaging one another, don't worry. You're still *in*, and you're earning *points* for your chivalry. So walk her to the door, or drive her home, and then…

-Read her.

I'm serious; this is the important part. Unless you're a complete write-off, you should have some indication of whether or not the goodnight kiss is going to happen.

You do NOT want to read this wrong. If you go in for the kill and she pulls away, whatever magic you might have made (suffering through God-awful movies) is dead.

Close your eyes, do *that sexy mouth thing* you've been working on, and, Lord willing, let her have it.

But please, please, please don't mess it up.

The ground you've gained tonight — be it an inch or a mile — is invaluable.

Who knows--

--next time *you* might even get to pick the movie.

How to Set Up that Second Date

Let's be honest—that first date was awkward as hell.

The whole time, you were *hoping to whoever you hope to* that the last piece of salad wasn't stuck to your teeth—and the movie after dinner wasn't easy, either.

Who can focus on a movie when they've got her sitting shotgun, right?

I mean, every time she yawns or stretches or brushes against you, you're reading into it
--hoping to whoever you hope to--
that you're taking her home tonight.

Okay, playboy, let's assume she's a *good* girl; let's assume your sorry ass went to bed alone and woke up wondering if *right now* is too soon to call her back.

Here's my first tip for setting up that second date;

right now *is* too soon to call her back.

Just like *everything else* about dating, there are unspoken rules to setting up another dinner, another movie, another *whatever*.

Rules to keep you from looking desperate.

Rules to keep you from appearing aggressive.

Rules to keep you from *blowing it.*

You will eventually; you're a guy, and blowing it is what we do. To keep you from blowing it right now, here's some rules to remember before picking up the phone.

1.) Grab your cell; put her number in speed dial.
You're going to be nervous when you dial; you don't want to call ten different digits by accident. By the time you get her number right, you'll be tired of being yelled at by Hungarian men with suspiciously similar voicemails.

2.) Don't panic when you get her on the line.
Remember, Romeo, if your date went reasonably well, she wants to see you again—sound casual, but speak with confidence when you tell her—

3.) —You want to do something *wild.*
'Wild' is in italics because 'wild' is important. 'Wild' is spontaneous,
'wild' is adventurous. 'Wild' is fun. 'Wild' is safe. Wild is *not* taking her to a swingers party just to show her how 'bad-ass' you are.

4.) Incorporate elements you learned on Date Number One. This is where you should have been paying attention, boys; everyone knows first dates are job interviews (--the job just happens to be sleeping together, or, at the very least, building the foundation of a prospective future relationship--) so hopefully you used *your* question of the inevitable *question-and-answer period* to learn important things; places she's never been, foods she's never tried, etc.

5.) For God's sake, show up on time.

Seriously, you'd be amazed how often we blow this one.

So, there you have it—a couple of fool-proof tips to engaging her interest in sitting across a table from you again.

If you need my help on dinner conversations, awkward pauses, or longing glances over candlelight—

--you may be better off alone.

The Art of Reconciliation

So maybe you see her at the mall.
Maybe you see her at the bar.

The restaurant, the trail, the market.
And all of a sudden *where* doesn't matter half as much as *who*.

Who is the one you let go; *who* is the one who got away.

She looks good, too—
--actually, she looked good when you had her, Romeo.

Now she's *beyond*.

So you're standing there, slack-jawed and broken hearted, and you're wondering how-in-the-hell you can make up for *whatever it is* you did to end it in the first place.

You're standing at the base of a mountain this time, boys; here are a couple of tips to make the *climb* easier.

-Don't apologize.

Not right away; don't get me wrong, you've got a lot of *"I'm sorry's"* ahead. But standing there, looking her in her beautiful blue or brown or green eyes, reminding her of what an asshole you are —
--not a good idea.

-Don't compliment her.

Excessively — anything more than "You look good" translates directly to "I-would-like-to-sleep-with-you-again."

-Don't push.

"Let's do dinner tomorrow" might be a little much. (Gauge this based on whether or not she slaps you after you say hello.)
Pump the brakes, playboy; maybe offer her your number; tell her you'd love to catch up over coffee *sometime*.
The key here is the 'sometime' — as in sometime of *her* choosing.

And then —
--take a breath —
--look her in her beautiful blue or brown or green eyes —
(Because if this doesn't work, you're about to let the best thing that ever happened to you walk away.)

(Again.)

--and say goodbye.

You read that right, guys—
--turn your sorry ass around, and let her go.

The *play* is that you hope you've peaked her interest.

You've showed her you've changed, you've grown; you've evolved from that Neanderthal you used to be.

You've created a little mystery, and, ideally, left her wondering what the hell is so fabulous that you would turn your back on her beautiful ass.

You're not atop the Himalayas yet, brave explorer; but, by the time she calls, you'll be a hell of a lot closer to the summit than the bottom.

How to Handle Your Raging Jealousy

I don't care how good looking you are.

I don't even care how good looking *you* think you are.

Your girlfriend looks *better*.

You realize this, of course; you must, even sub-consciously, notice that every time you two are at the mall, or at dinner, or the movies, or *anywhere*, really, where other people are—

--she gets more attention than you do.

Now, this might awaken your macho sense of competition—and don't get me wrong—if trying to keep up to her means you iron your T-Shirts every now and then, I'm all for it.

If you take it too far, however—if you take it out on her—then maybe she should realize what you've secretly known all along.

She could do better.

It's harsh, boys: this is the reality we live in. We're all attention-whores, in our own little ways — but the amount of us that be-little, or degrade, or demean our women — just to make ourselves feel better — *astronomical*.

You boil every little comment, or indiscretion, or lie down to its essence: your bruised ego is the reason you fly off the handle.

So man up, and read on: here are some sure-fire ways to recognizing she's the best (without admitting defeat.)

-Value her status in the relationship. She's your *partner*, Douchebag; not something you bring with you to a restaurant when you're hungry. Behind those perfectly shaped eyes sitting across the table are perfectly shaped *opinions*, values, and ideals.

Spend time gazing into *them*, instead of scanning the surrounding diners for other men (with or without their tongues hanging out.)

-Value *your* status in the relationship. God, or evolution, or *her parents* created the vision that you happen to be dating; and, for thousands and thousands of years, women have been objects of desire, lust and beauty. For thousands and thousands of years, guys like you have chased them.

Not the other way around.

That's just how it works, fellas.

-She's with you for a reason. (This ties into valuing your status in the relationship.)

Don't bother trying to figure out just what that reason is.

I can't either.

-Understand that, while she looks good in a dress
--or a skirt—
--or jeans—
--or anything at all, really—

--she has just as many messed up insecurities and problems as you do. Maybe more. (It's hard out there for the ladies.)

So if, by chance, she can walk into a room with her chin up, and her hips *out*, the confidence she exudes is to be *commended*, not questioned.

In closing, while I appreciate your need to be the one-and-only *worshipper at her alter*, I recommend you take the cat calls, sideways looks (and occasional whistles) in stride. The more…enlightened…of us even view these as compliments.

Remember, she *is* gorgeous, jackass — that's why you asked her out in the first place.

So the next time you two are following the waiter to your table, enjoy the looks she's (most definitely) getting.

Chances are, she's going home with you tonight.

And that, boys, is as close to winning as we're *ever* going to get.

How to Meet Her Mother

It's the most terrifying thing you'll ever do.

Well, *second* most terrifying, *maybe* — but meeting her father is a whole 'nother ballgame, and therefore a whole 'nother article.

And you know, don't you, that from the second she lays eyes on you, she's judging you.

Examining you.

Determining your worth.

Trying to figure out — much the way *you* have been — if you're the guy for her precious little girl.

Good luck, fellas.

Look, this is one particular minefield I can't steer you through — just as every woman is a *precious, unique snowflake*; every woman's mother is a precious, unique snow *storm*, waiting to unleash her fury upon you.

All I can do to protect you is arm you with the knowledge that, should you defy expectations and rise above *hers*, a good mother will welcome you into her (extended) family with open arms.

There is sunshine at the end of this one boys—here's how to hang in there.

The scenario: a friendly get-together over *brunch*—a Mother's favorite meal.

-Accept the fact that, *somewhere*, in her illustrious dating past, your girl dated a man who was probably twice (at least in Ma's eyes) the man Ma figures *you* are.

Now, don't let this get you down. She just met you. You've got *minutes*—or however long you're meeting with Ma for—to convince her otherwise.

-Mothers hate showboating.

I don't care if you're the CEO of a *Fortune-500* company; if you're meeting her mother over brunch, and Mom offers to pay, let her. Or resist, *once*, calmly—and keep your voice barely above a whisper.

She's trying to *bait* you—to see if you're going to grandstand about being able to 'provide for her baby girl.' (And you may very well *have been* for the duration of the relationship—but I'll wager she's been providing for a lot longer than that, hotshot.)

-Mothers like manners.

Meaning that, yeah, it's okay to pick up the check (-- as long as she doesn't resist.) Do it discreetly.

-I know that there's some blonde over in the other booth who keeps eyeing you.

On any other occasion, you may be foolish enough to believe you can steal a lingering gaze or two, unbeknownst to your lady.

This is not 'any other occasion.'

I don't care how hot the blonde is, or how daft you (incorrectly) assume your girl is—her mother will catch you.

Hell, she *wants* you to look.

Because she wants to catch you.

-Her Mother was once wooed herself.

This is important to remember; although she's the obstacle right now, the beautiful lady across the table—*the one who birthed the beautiful lady beside you*—was once charmed also.

Blood from a stone, boys.

Blood from a stone.

Finally, and probably paramount:

Once again—

--the beautiful lady across the table

birthed the beautiful lady beside you.

So no matter how meeting her Mother goes—

--she's already done you a *solid.*

How to Let Her Go

You love her, right?

Not just the way she makes you feel —

--or the things she does for you —

you genuinely, deeply, really-*really* love the girl.

You're just not *in* love anymore, and that's okay.

There are ways to let her go, without losing her forever — ways to give you both the space you *probably* need (--probably, because, if she's a good girl, there's a very good chance you're making a mistake.)

-Tell her the truth.
  I know, fellas — this seems weird; you're wondering if it would be better to sugar-coat it.
  Let's face it; *'I'm not in love with you anymore'* doesn't sound good.
  It hurts.
  It *should*.
  You're leaving her — hard enough — the least you can do is be a *man* about it.

-Tell her the truth somewhere she feels comfortable.

You don't want to *sandbag* her—taking her out to your favorite restaurant—your *very*

public favorite restaurant—not a good place to induce tears.

(It's the equivalent of setting up the pins, and then throwing a strike.)

-Leave the door open.

No, that doesn't mean keep her number in your phone for drunken-booty calls at 3 am.

She's going to be vulnerable. Do NOT take advantage of this.

One day, soon, she's *not* going to vulnerable, and she'll remember what a dick you are.

-Give her time.

She needs to get over you (--it's not as hard as you think--) which means girl-talk and nights out and nights in and *nights without you.*

You wanted this, stud-muffin.

Deal with it.

-After giving the appropriate amount of time, call her.

Again, this is not to 'hook up.' This is to see, genuinely, how she feels.

If you genuinely don't care how she feels, then you skip this step.

(And again, she's probably better off without you.)

-Take time for yourself.

Not binge drinking and playing fantasy football—those are things you were probably lucky enough to do (on occasion) when you were with her. No, take time to evaluate what you want out of a relationship, and just what it was about her that made you believe it couldn't work in the first place.

-Have a good cry.

It's coming, fellas—sooner or later, amidst all of this, you're going to believe (correctly or incorrectly) that you've thrown away the best thing that ever happened to you.

You probably have.

You're an idiot.

Deep breath—we're *all* idiots.

-Beg her to take you back.

And, next time, think before you open your mouth.

The grass is greener and all that.

After all;

You love her, right?

Not just the way she makes you feel—

--or the things she does for you—

you genuinely, deeply, really-*really* love the girl.

Good girls are hard to come by;

foolish boys, (unfortunately for us--)

--*not so much.*

How to Meet Her Father

It's the most terrifying thing you'll ever do.

For real this time.

Because this time, you're not meeting her mother.

No, Romeo; you're meeting her *Daddy*.

Here's how to survive.

First of all, realize that, *yes*, it's Daddy. Not 'Father,' not 'Sir (--well, to *you*, he's sir, but to her--)

Yeah.

Daddy.

Which means she's Daddy's Little Girl—which means you're the guy who's taking her away.

Which means you're the bad guy.

Fellas, this is okay—just remember, when you're shaking his hand (and trying to shake it as hard as he is--) and when you're trying to look him in the eyes (--because you know he's looking into yours--) that, someday, you're going to have a daughter of your own.

And that someday, some jackass is going to take her away from you.

All of a sudden, (--probably as he's crushing your hand—) you can see where the big guy is coming from.

This has nothing to do with age, either—whether you're fifteen or thirty-five (and, hopefully, she's in the *ballpark*; otherwise, you're *screwed*) any Dad worth his salt will react to meeting you the exact same way.

Call it '*guarded optimism*;' sure, right now, (--as you're trying to regain the feeling in your fingers--) the look on his face says '*I'm gonna kill you*.'

Trust me, deep down, he's hoping you're the guy who's gonna treat her right.

(You can't blame him if '*The-guy-who-made-her-cry-senior-year*' and '*The-guy-who-left-her-in-a-bodega-in-Mexico*' are flashing across his subconscious as you tell him you've only got the best intentions for his baby.)

Remember this, and you're halfway home.

Now, let's say you're invited into the living room (--or the corner booth at *Daddy's Little Girl's* favorite restaurant--) to formally introduce yourself. This is the 'job interview' portion of the meeting; and there are definitely some topics you want to discuss—and some you want to *avoid*.

-Playing 'Johnny-Big-Wheel'=murder.
No, it doesn't matter that you make 60k a year, and that you're investment portfolio is '*promising*.'

He's her father.

This means he makes *more* than you. And if, by some miracle, he *doesn't*—you damn well better *pretend* he does.

-Reminiscing about your glory days means *you don't have any left.* Sure, you were *All-State* back in the day. While I can appreciate the attempt to butter him up with sports stories, the only words to come out of your (probably-unworthy) mouth are better suited for praising *Daddy's Little Girl.*

-On the topic of sports: if his favorite team comes up in conversation, you damn well better admit that you like *Said Team.*

Even if *Said Team* sucks.

Even if *Said Team* are *your* team's division rivals, and even if admitting you like *Said Team* kills you a little inside.

He's her father.

He could kill you, more than a *little*, and more than *inside*.

(*The exception to this, of course, is if said team is the Indianapolis Colts. They suck so hard, they're beyond defending.)

Make no mistake about it; meeting her father is like going to war. Only, (hopefully,) without the wanton destruction and needless atrocities.

The best way to come out alive (--because, as in war, nobody comes out unscathed--) is to bow your admittedly unworthy head, acquiesce to his superiority, and admit that, *despite the Colts*, you have one thing in common.

You both love *Daddy's Little Girl.*

It won't win you the war—but, if you really mean it—you may live to fight another day.

How to Get Over Yourself

You spend more time in front of the mirror than your girl does.

It's okay to admit it; she's known for a while, and she still puts up with you. Really, it's just one of your *many* shortcomings, right fellas? You leave dishes out, you're chronically late (--or obsessively early ;) you tend to miss days between showers.

And still, somehow, you're able to delude yourself into believing you're *the man*.

You believe — somewhere deep, deep down — somewhere you go in moments of crushing insecurity — that, should your lady leave, you'll be able to find another.

Somebody as beautiful as her; someone as intelligent as her, someone (most importantly) as patient as her.

You're wrong.

What we, as a group — and to a man — need to realize — is that if we're fortunate enough to have a good woman in our lives, we're plenty lucky enough.

We don't need to be in the mirror as much as we are.

Hell, we don't need to be in the bar as much as we are, either.

What we should be doing — as a group, and to a man — is thanking whatever-deity-we-choose-to-thank that we're lucky enough to hold down a woman who is probably better off without us.

We should be spending more time cooking dinners.

We should be spending more time showing up for the dinners they cook for us.

We should be avoiding the bars, and the pick-up games, and the million-and-two *other* things we focus on, when we're deluded into believing they'll put up with us either way.

When we're deluded into believing we're *the man*, and that if she goes — finally having had enough of whatever it is we focus on *instead* of her — we'll find someone comparable.

We won't.

See, there really is nothing more comforting to us — as a group, and to a man — than knowing some girl is at home, waiting to hear about our triumphs and defeats.

Waiting to console us when we need it; to be there for us when we're foolish enough to believe we *don't*.

Waiting to be the *source* of the feeling that puts us in front of the mirror — the source that forces that smile on our faces.

The source that deludes us — as a group, and to a man — into believing we're THE man.

Because, really, it's all because — and all for — *them* anyways.

So the next time you're in front of the mirror — or off to the bar, or the pickup game — reconsider the *reason* you're so damned confident —

--and thank her for putting up with you in the first place.

The Art of 'Spicing it Up'

You can't stand it when she leaves her makeup on the counter.

When she overcooks the lasagna.

When she lets the dog on your Grandmother's couch; when she wakes up on the wrong side of the bed.

When she looks at you cock-eyed.

Hell, you're frustrated by just about everything.

What you fail to realize—what you so very desperately *need* to realize—is that your frustrations really have nothing to do with her, at all.

You're in a rut, superstar.

And you're projecting your frustrations, your inadequacies, and your anxieties onto her.

Now, before you panic—just as the light bulb in your brain goes off—

--relax.

We all do this from time to time.

We're men, after all.

The solution, obviously, starts (--as you probably figure most things do--) with you.

Specifically, how you view her.

The everyday things—the lasagna, the dog and Grandma's couch—signify that you need to shake things up; to get away from the routine you've fallen into, and the focus it has made you put on the (perceived) shortcomings of your partner.

A couple of dates outside your comfort zone will have you viewing her in a different light, as you re-discover (--or discover--) aspects about her you forgot or failed to see before.

Say you like going to the movies.

Screw
The
Movies.

Take her rock climbing instead.

Say you love a picnic in the park (--and yes, it's okay to admit that--)

--bet you'd love a picnic on a rented sailboat even more.

Say, (--because you will, initially--) that you don't have the capital to be making wild, extravagant plans right now. Say the last quarter hit you harder than Billy in seventh grade, and your budget is tighter than the drawstring on her track-pants.

Loosen them up with creative, inexpensive dates.

A weekend away, but at a bed-and-breakfast instead of the Hilton.

Zip-lining a cave instead of swimming with dolphins.

Bottom line, there are options out there; best of all, your creativity will yield unexpected results, and help you to see other aspects of your partner.

Who knows—maybe she'll even get over the million things she dislikes about *you*.

Getting the Right Gift

Birthdays. Anniversaries. Christmas.

These are *Hallmark* days we're living in; there's an occasion for everything.

I don't care if you've been with her for ten weeks or ten years:
When one of those occasions rolls around, it's on you to find the right gift.

Not necessarily the prettiest, shiniest, or most expensive gift.

The *right* gift.

To a man, we're still just as dumbfounded at the concept of shopping for the fairer sex as we've ever been — if not *more*.

Not necessarily *dumb*, fellas —

--dumbfounded.

After all, there's an etiquette to buying *that-certain-something* — these days, there's just as many rules for gift giving as there are days that (unofficially, of course) demand it.

Here's a couple tips on surviving 'till the next occasion.

-Hold back a little.

Sure, you've been with her for three months, and now, *finally*, that first *birthday-anniversary-special occasion-just-because* has rolled around. You want to impress her. You want to floor her, to send her giggling hysterically to her next coffee date with her *just-as-impressed* friends.

Don't.

You're setting the bar here, guys — although she may not realize it (--unless she's one in a million, in which case: marry her already--) this random (though still somewhat expected) act of kindness sets the bar for all of your *other* random acts of kindness to follow.

So put the credit card down, hotshot.

You've got plenty more chances to whip it out ahead.

-Christmas is coming.

Sometime within the next 365 days, anyways.

This ties into the previous point—while it's positively amazing that you spoil her on occasion (-- and she *does* deserve it--) you have to remember that, in this consumer-driven society, Christmas is the Motherload of 'occasions.'

And it's coming.

Plan accordingly.

-Do it for the right reasons.

Getting laid is fun. And important (to us, anyways.)

It is not a reason to treat her to something special.

-It's not about the cost.

Stop laughing, fellas. It's true. If you take the time to make her something, or, *heaven forbid,* use your head and come up with something clever to get her — something that reminds her of a time you shared, or a special moment together — it'll mean more than some random, thoughtless bauble.

Regardless of *said random baubles'* cost.

For the most part.

So there you have it — it's all about the *thought* behind the gift (behind the occasion.)

Put some effort into it — make it mean something — hell, make it mean something to both of you — and the dividends are great.

If you're lucky, they might just be greater than the standard you've now set for yourself.

...

The Meathead Manifesto, Book 3

Meditations on Nutrition…and Supplementation (…and other stuff I'm grossly unqualified to give advice on.)

Protein Intake (For Meatheads)

For every article championing the benefits of mass protein consumption, there are two more damning the concept.

Musclemags and meatheads will tell you to shoot for one gram of protein for every pound you *want* to weigh:

If you're shooting for a lean, chiseled one-sixty-five, you should strive for one hundred and sixty-five grams of protein, per day.

If, on the other hand, you're aiming to bulk up — you better pump up your intake. Two hundred twenty-five grams of the good stuff might seem obscene at first; remember to supplement your diet with powders, shakes, and food sources of all kinds.

Variety will keep you from pulling your hair out when reaching for the sixtieth chicken breast of the week.

Remember, these are guidelines for serious gainers only—there have been studies claiming that any more than 20g of protein is indigestible at any time—and that the excess is stored as fat.

However, if you're crushing it out at the gym on a daily basis—and I know you are—then you're gonna need plenty of fuel to recover from those incline presses.

And, if you need any more proof as to the validity of mass-consumption—download *Pumping Iron*, and watch Arnold and the boys from *Gold's* order breakfast.

Protein Intake for Girly-Men (and Girls!!)

The other side of the argument (as relates to ideal levels of protein consumption) states that, for the most part, bodybuilders and gym-bunnies tend to over-do it.

I know, I know—the culture predominately associated with obsessive, repetitive acts of self-destruction (*and reconstruction*!) might-maybe push the boundaries of 'healthy' eating.

There are studies claiming, as I've mentioned, that excess protein is simply excreted (*eew*) or stored as fat. (*EWW*)

While meatheads like myself don't believe in excess (--hence, proudly, why we're meatheads) even the most body-conscious of us recognize the counter-productiveness of packing on *unwanted* pounds.

So, if your goal is weight loss *or* weight-control—*or* anything other than weight-gain, really, then you *still* need protein.

You just need to monitor *how much.*

Any kind of exercise requires rest and nutrients to recover from—the majority of documentation suggests protein, carbohydrate, and even fat play a role here.

Protein sources vary wildly—many think of whey mixtures when picturing that post-workout shake. Casein, soy, and even (gasp) food sources offer similar nutritional content (as outlined in the next fabulous chapter.)

So grab the protein of your choice; and whether you're mixing with water or milk or goat's blood, shoot for 20g per serving.

Remember, a mix of protein and carbs an hour before lift-off (*pun*) can do wonders for your workout.
Another serving, within an hour of finishing may be the most important (--take that, breakfast) meal of the day.

Whey vs. Casein vs. Soy vs. Food vs. You.

Whey is mother's milk for meatheads.
It *builds* stuff.

Casein is whey's naughty little neighbor.
A little lighter, great just before bed.

Soy is a healthy alternative for vegetarians, dairy-haters, and hipsters.

Food has protein. Eat it.
Usually, high protein foods contain 2.5% protein by weight.

You are sexy when you're learning.

A Final Meditation on Protein

The amount that you actually digest and absorb (or *bioavailability*) is wholly dependent on you; how well your guts are working, what you've consumed that day, etc.

Little hint: Diarrhea means you've overdone it.

Caffeine is Good for You!!!!

Let that sink in for a minute; I realize it goes against conventional wisdom.
The rule of thumb has long been *"If it tastes good, then it's bad for you."*

And while this is usually the case (damn you, Cheeseburgers) the fact of the matter is that coffee is a cheap, effective supplement, if used correctly.

A cup before exercise can do wonders for your energy levels; ten cups before will have your training partner thinking you're railing lines in the parking lot.

Sugar is the main bad guy here. We tend to over-indulge—hell, it takes a mountain to make most drive-thru blends tolerable.
Studies have linked sugar intake to hypoglycemia, and it may contribute (directly or indirectly) to diabetes and obesity.

Not cool, if you're trying to maintain any kind of physique.
In moderation, the benefits of caffeine for both bodybuilders and shapers can be summed in one glorious word:

Adrenaline.

It's that kick in the pants, that shot to the central nervous system that makes Tuesday *TUESDAY!!!!*
And leg day *LEG DAY!!!!*

Also, dopamine. The chemical in your brain that pushes the 'pleasure' button. The one you like so very, very much during sex. That euphoria runners claim to feel during a marathon (--something I have no clue about.)
Apparently, it also helps with endurance, if you're lacking. (I wouldn't know anything about that, either.)

You're addicted to the stuff anyway—you might as well feel good about it.

Creatine is Not the Enemy.

We need fuel.

For walking the dog.
For yelling at the neighbors when they tell you to clean up after the dog.
For bench pressing three-hundred pounds three-hundred times.

Our fuel is (deep breath) Adenosine Triphosphate. (ATP.) I could bore you to tears with the bio-chemistry of it all; all you need to realize is that we use three mechanisms to produce ATP.

The *best* is 'Creatine Kinase' — notice the word *Creatine* in there. This bad-boy is responsible for every gut-check bicep curl we do.

Say you're on the squat rack. Every rep costs ATP, which converts to Adenosine Diphosphate (ADP — acronyms are fun!!) as you lower yourself into the squat — and ADP is useless.
If you're full of Creatine, it lends the missing letters of the alphabet to ADP, turning your *D* back into *T* (by lending a phosphate — or something) and letting you finish the rep.

So, it stands to reason that the more you've got in your system, the harder you'll lift!

Food sources, like meats and fish, are full of the stuff, although a great deal is lost in the cooking process.

And, since most of us only store 60-80% of our potential Creatine levels, supplementation is an effective boost.

How much hasn't been locked down yet; some bodybuilders supplement with pre-workout meals, and post-workout shakes.

(Unless) Creatine is the Enemy.

Since its rise to dominance in the supplement wars, Creatine has had a fair share of detractors. Much of the bad press stems from the product's alleged side-effects.

Reports of muscle, ligament & tendon strains (as a result of Superman-esque muscle contractions) have been supposedly caused by Creatine supplementation.

As the theory goes, Billy Bodybuilder, arms full of Creatine, can contract (squeeze) <u>so</u> <u>hard</u> at the top of a preacher curl, that both muscle cells and connective tissues *explode* under the strain of his mighty flex.

Creatine, by improving the explosive energy output of Billy's guns, overwhelms the actual existing mechanical strength of the muscle itself; the result is ripping and tearing and sobbing.

Lots of sobbing.
Now, there are no studies proving this—and it stands to reason that Billy might be pushing harder, due to the *perceived* 'boost' he feels the supplement has given him—but it is worth noting, nonetheless.

Most problems stemming from supplementation are strictly dosage related. Stomach cramping and diarrhea at the gym aren't fun; to avoid them, follow the instruction label on the bottle — always.

If there is a 'loading phase' (where you're taking a ton, in comparison to the regular 'maintenance phase') be sure to scale back when instructed to do so.

Many a gym-hero has adopted the *'more-is-more'* mentality, and taken the max dosage, for the maximum duration; this in turn could cause maximum strain on the kidneys...and the toilet seat.

Steroids are bad.

Backne.

That is all.

Carbs are fun!

Face it; there are more diet guides out there than there are pretty-dirty-pretty girls at your local *Hooters*.

Some tell you to cut carbs, some tell you to carbo-*load*; some tell you to only eat carbs on the third Monday of the month. (Since pretty much every single thing we put into our mouths contains carbohydrate, this last one can be tricky.)

Remember that bit before about Adenosine Triphosphate (ATP) being fuel for our bodies? Well, ATP is created by glucose, which we in turn receive from…*dun dun dun*…carbohydrate.

What it all means is, if you've got a goal—any ideal shape or weight in mind—you're gonna need carbs.

Lots of 'em.

Bar none, these bad-boys are the most important energy source for working muscles, as well as things us meatheads *sometimes* use.
Like brains.
(And central nervous systems.)

Now, there are two types of carbs—*simple* (sugars like those in jam, or fruit) and *complex* (pasta, bread, cereal.)

Unfortunately, we tend to get much of our simple carb content from the added sugars in soda and bad drive-thru rather than, say, fruit.

Complex carbs are best consumed with veggies, fruits, dairy and whole grains, since they're packed with vitamins, and minerals, and other stuff that sounds good for you.

And since one gram of carbohydrate equals (only!) four calories, you can get plenty in a day without feeling like you're making drastic changes to your diet.

Shoot for 45-65% of your total daily caloric intake, and you're getting enough carbs to fuel that workout you're busting tomorrow morning.

Fat, like the stuff you need (as opposed to the thing that you think you are.)

You need it.
In your diet, not your *ass*.

Some of you are probably on some ridiculous diet right now, snacking on raindrops and generally feeling horrible.

Why?
You need fat.

The good stuff (preferably *un*saturated) is rammed with essential fatty acids—essential (key word) fatty acids that produce essential little things like cell-membranes. And hormones.

You like clear skin?
Eat fat.

Feeling full after meals? (I'm looking at you, raindrops.)
Eat fat.

Being packed with vitamins A, D, E, K and sexy?
Fat.

To give you a little guideline as to how much, remember there are 9 calories in every gram. Toss this number into your daily cal-counter (chances are you've got one) and you have an idea of just how much you need on a daily basis.

20-35% of your daily intake of calories (total) should be from fat—good stuff like fish, nuts and olive oil. Stay the hell away from hydrogenated fats, fast food, and most of the fried stuff.

I'm not telling you to stop scoping the fat content on the side of the label (I do it too;) I'm simply suggesting that the next time you read the word *'fat'* beside *'it's-what's-for-dinner'* that you don't run screaming for the toilet.

The Paleo Diet (Or, Your Excuse to Eat like the Caveman You Are)

We're always looking for that *next* thing: the superfood that can cure cancer, the vitamin to reverse the aging process, the diet that can cure our collective obesity.

Somewhere along the line in our search for the future, we decided it best to look back.

Way back.

And so the latest trend in 'surefire-ways-to-become-better' isn't really anything new—it's roughly 2.5 million years old.

The Stone Age is where we've gone searching for answers: The Paleolithic Period, to be exact; hence the Paleo, 'hunter-gatherer' diet.

Overlooking the benefits the advent of agriculture has borne, Paleo suggests that our genomes haven't changed much in the past 500 generations, and that, as a result, we're better off maintaining the diet (and lifestyle!) of the Stone Age.

Before you go club/drag the next beautiful woman to your cave, consider this:

Going Paleo means excluding processed foods (of any kind) as well as added sugars and salts.

Tolerable, right?

Interestingly, grains of all kinds get the axe, along with dairy (!) beans, lentils and legumes.

The kicker—

--alcohol has to go, too.

(Well, let's cap it off at three drinks/week, anyways…we have to be realistic.)

Foods included in the Caveman Diet:

Grass-fed meats and game, wild fish, eggs, unprocessed fruits and vegetables, nuts (except for peanuts) seeds and some oils. (eg. Olive oil, Macadamia.)

The reasoning behind going Stone Age? Archeological studies suggest little to no cardiovascular disease existed in the time of our ancestors, despite the high-meat diet. Conversely, many (--the argument could be made for pretty much all--) of our diseases and disorders could be traced to the advent of agriculture; everything from cancer to heart disease to joint disorders to acne.

Bold claims, to be sure; however evidence exists connecting acid/base balance to any and all health conditions. Naturally, studies and arguments offering conflicting information exist on any recommended diet, as well...always take the information with a proverbial grain of salt.

Advocates recommend adherence to the Caveman Diet 85% of the time, with three 'open' meals per week (--as is the standard for a pretty much all 'diets.')

Basing their claims on the fact that, while we have evolved on a plethora of different food consumption modalities, a common thread over the centuries has been the lack of processed foods, added sugars and salts—so why include them in our diet today?

Protein—long acknowledged as the cornerstone of the meathead meal—is satiating and helps support muscle mass and immune system function. Naturally, a protein-rich diet, like Paleo, tends to control weight and glycemic level.

Perhaps the most beneficial aspect of the plan, however, comes from the assurances that fats are not as bad as once perceived; consuming Omega-3 rich foods, in particular, are benchmarks of the Paleo plan.

In terms of omitted foods—sure, grains, dairy, and legumes may not be essential elements of all diets— however, do we really need to axe them altogether?

Implementing elements of the Paleo Diet—the emphasis on lean protein sources, the omission of processed foods and the illumination on 'healthy' fats—are well worth consideration; as with everything, however, until conclusive research exists, full-on adherence should be carefully scrutinized.

*To be fair, only one randomized, controlled trial regarding the effects and benefits of the Paleo diet method has been performed—many more would be required before an accurate conclusion can be ascertained.

6 is more than 3.

And six is how many meals I want you eating tomorrow, six because six is more than three.

More is more, and it's my motto; not only because it's awesome and I'm a meathead, but because, in this case, more is *actually* better.

And not just in my little fantasy world.

The fact is, if you eat six meals, evenly spaced, throughout the course of your day, not only will you have more energy (as the supply is readily available in your system,) but you'll eat smaller portions per sitting.

That feeling of satiation will keep your tummy from rumbling, which will keep you from embarrassing yourself in front of your co-workers, which will keep you from crying in that buffet line you'll inevitably hit on the way home.

Not only that, but your metabolism will be running hotter than South Beach on Saturday, (so very hot) keeping you burning excess calories, and ensuring you've got plenty of fuel for both workouts and weekends.

I realize that, initially, this can be a difficult concept to grasp.

"But I want to lose weight, and you're telling me to eat more?" is one of the things I hear most in the gym, right after

"But my husband is out of town all weekend." (--This may or may not be in my little fantasy world.)

We were intended (by Zeus, the All-Father) to be grazers, and our digestive systems are designed as such. It's science.

Fasting plays havoc on our bodies—skipping meals (in an effort to lose weight) causes our metabolism to slow to a crawl, as our bodies store fat, not knowing when we'll get the nutrients contained within next. Therefore, remember six > three.

Going Gluten Free

Gluten, a storage protein found in wheat, barley and rye has been linked to Celiac disease. (Celiac is an autoimmune disease 'whereby villi of the small intestine are destroyed by the presence of even trace amounts of gluten' in the diet.)

Estimated to affect one in every one-hundred-thirty-three individuals, evidence suggests the reported cases of Celiac disease will continue to rise.

Symptoms include gastrointestinal distress, fatigue, reduced iron stores, headaches and joint pain. The disease is diagnosed by blood tests, followed by a small bowel biopsy: to date, the only treatment for Celiac disease is adherence to a strict, gluten-free diet *for life*.

As recently as 2012, *Fasano et al.* proposed the term *"Gluten-Sensitivity"* to encompass non-Celiac immune-mediated response to gluten. Meaning, in layman's terms, a whole hell of a lot of us (-- estimated at six percent of the current world population--) are at least somewhat intolerant to Gluten, if not suffering from Celiac. Though the symptoms of sensitivity present similar to Celiac disease, a sensitivity will not elicit a positive Celiac screen…unfortunately, no validated medical test to detect gluten sensitivity exists.

Some theorists, including Dr. William Davis, in his 2011 book *Wheat Belly*, claim modern wheat is partly (--perhaps even largely--) responsible for most diseases in modern civilization; including but not limited to obesity, heart disease, cancer, Type 2 diabetes, arthritis, Alzheimer's—as well as the aforementioned Celiac.

Wheat, rye and barley have been staples of the human diet for thousands of years—why the shift from sustenance to shunned?

Theorists like Davis argue that today's wheat has been genetically altered to become increasingly drought-resistant, and to produce greater yields...farms today produce *ten times* the yield of those but a few generations prior. Such changes have significantly changed the genetic code of the wheat itself; the result—we simply are not eating the same food our ancestors did.

(*And, given that the human digestive system hasn't evolved that much in the past couple-million years, we're a little slow to adapt to wildly different sources.)

Without delving into the mind-numbing science of it all; sometime in the 1940's the 'International Maize and Wheat Improvement Centre' was founded outside Mexico City in an effort to reduce hunger by imposing yields of wheat, corn and soy.

Good idea, right?

A Geneticist by the name of Dr. Norman Borlaug helped develop 'Dwarf wheat;' a veritable super-wheat—albeit a super-wheat with a much, much higher gluten content.

Regardless of the validity of modern wheat's contribution, there is no denying that Gluten-sensitivity—if not outright Celiac disease—is all too common in today's population.

While no scientific data exists suggesting a Gluten-free diet will result in weight loss, the argument can certainly be made that limiting intakes of grain-based foods will play a role in any fat-loss program one might adapt.

Meathead meal plan: For days ending in 'y.'

Breakfast:
Carb, protein-heavy mix, with a splash of fat on the side.
Also, sunshine.

Go for egg whites—hell, treat yourself to the whole egg—with some whole wheat toast. Coffee is the key ingredient here.

Mid-morning snack:
Veggies (spinach and vinegar, for your forearms!)
Lean chicken breast, salad.
Tuna (little secret—mix with pineapple chunks. Cuts the smell, makes the taste tolerable!)

Before workout:
Lean turkey breast sammich, salmon, almonds.

Workout:
Iron.
(Get it?)

Post workout:
Up to 40g whey protein, for hard-gainers, with some carbs.

20g protein, if you're looking to maintain, or slim down. Choose whey or soy, or food source.

Dinner:
Pasta (go whole wheat with the noodles, remember you still need fiber, and carbs!)
Salad with chicken or turkey, fish, a healthy stir-fry.

Before bed:
Protein, because your muscles will be repairing themselves   overnight.
Casein (slow digesting protein) is a great choice here, as whey is absorbed into the system very quickly, and you'll need a supply of nutrients the course of your sleep.

Oatmeal can be a good choice here as well.

A Final Bit of Advice (in lieu of an epilogue)

By now, if you've read even a *fraction* of the articles in '*The Meathead Manifesto,*' you're well on your way to being the Undisputed Heavyweight Champ.

The champ of women and girls—girl's fathers, and their expectations; the champ of lifting heavy things (many times in a row) and the champ of proper nutritional supplementation.

The heavyweight title is a *heavy* one, and the knowledge you've attained here makes you the omnipotent (--look it up) master of your gym, bedroom, kitchen, basement—hell, you're The Man, *everywhere* you go, now.

So go on—enjoy being the boss, but remember, the line between 'educated meathead' and 'entitled douchebag' is a thin one; use the information contained within these pages responsibly.

www.ingramcontent.com/pod-product-compliance
Lightning Source LLC
Chambersburg PA
CBHW032138020426
42334CB00016B/1210